Graves' Disease and Hyperthyroidism

Questions and Answers

By

Shunzhong Shawn Bao, MD

Editor: Barbara Winter

Ace Health Publisher

Publisher's Note/Disclaimer

The information contained herein is not intended to replace the services of a trained health professional or to be a substitute for individual medical advice. You should consult with your healthcare professional regarding any matter related to your health, and in particular, any matter that may require diagnosis and medical attention.

First Edition 2018

Graves' Disease and Hyperthyroidism

Questions and Answers
Shunzhong Shawn Bao, MD
Barbara Winter, Editor

Published by Ace Health Publisher

Dedication

This book is dedicated to my patients. These are their intelligent questions for which I am grateful. They motivate me to think, continue learning and improving my patient care every day. These days, doctors do not have enough time to address all the questions patients may have. I hope my patients will get some answers here.

I want to thank my nurses, Betty Westbury and Walter Chavis who are providing excellent care to my patients and were the first readers of this book. With their critiques, they have made significant contributions.

This book is also dedicated to my good friend, my editor, Barbara Winter, for her unending kindness and generosity. With her patience and critical editing, she has made this book readable.

Finally, this book is dedicated to my wife who deserves deep, enduring gratitude, and also to my two children who are both in medical school. They are "first round editors". They helped me despite their heavy medical school work. They inspire me to learn and strive for excellence in patient care.

Preface

Graves' disease is a relatively uncommon condition. When people hear this diagnosis their first reaction is "what is that?" People are also confused about Graves' disease, hyperthyroidism, and thyrotoxicosis. In this book I answer questions like these and also questions about possible causes and available treatments. In addition, I address questions about diet and its relationship to hyperthyroidism.

This book is not just to help you understand different kinds of hyperthyroidism and but also discusses how and why we treat them. Sometimes, the condition is straightforward, and sometimes, it can be very complicated.

While providing very practical guidelines for patients, this book addresses specific questions such as how to prepare for some common thyroid tests, how to prepare for thyroid surgery, how to prepare for radioactive iodine treatment, how to take thyroid medications, etc. Diet is also an important part of hyperthyroidism. I have one chapter devoted to it.

Patients with Graves' disease and hyperthyroidism or who have a family history of thyroid conditions, as well as those who just want to learn more about the disease will all benefit from reading this book and keeping it as a reference.

Contents

Chapter 1. The Basics of the Thyroid and Diagnosis of Graves' Disease and Hyperthyroidism

What is the thyroid?

The term "Thyroid gland" is derived from the Latin Glandula Thyreoidea meaning "shield-shaped gland". It is located at the base of your neck.

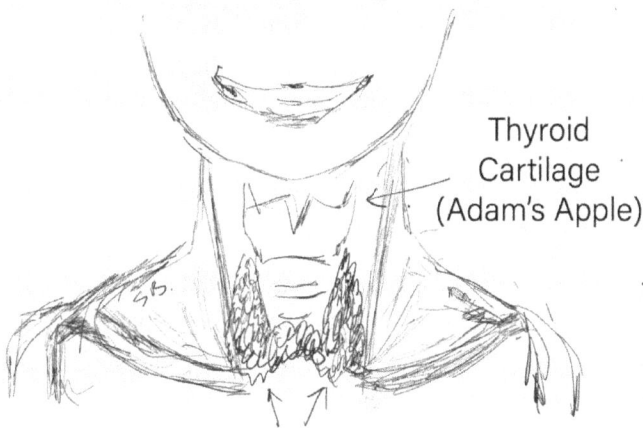

Thyroid
Cartilage
(Adam's Apple)

Thyroid Lobes

Fig. Illustration of thyroid gland at the base of neck (by Dr. Bao).

The thyroid hormones are T3 and T4. T3 is the active hormone that affects every cell, every tissue, or organ in our body. It is crucial for cells to function properly.

What is Graves' disease?

Graves' disease was named after the famous Irish surgeon, Robert James Graves (March 27, 1796 – March 20, 1853). Graves' disease is an autoimmune disease. Antibodies act on thyroid cells (thyrocytes) as thyrotropin hormone stimulating thyroid hormone synthesis and secretion as well as thyroid growth (causing a diffuse goiter). Antibodies can also cause eye disease (orbitopathy), and occasionally a skin rash/swelling-dermopathy referred to as pretibial or localized myxedema.

Some people spell Graves' disease as Grave's disease which is wrong. The Irish surgeon's last name was Graves, not Grave.

Some students call all hyperthyroidism Graves' disease which is also wrong. Graves' disease only refers to the cluster of conditions which are caused by autoimmune problems. There are many causes of hyperthyroidism.

How do you diagnose Graves' disease?

I make the diagnosis of Graves' disease based on the clinical presentation and lab tests. Most Graves' disease patients have extra thyroidal symptoms besides an overactive thyroid, such as eye disease, pretibial or localized myxedema.

A lab test revealing an overactive thyroid is important. A positive result of TSI (thyroid stimulating immunoglobulin) is the diagnostic test.

How many thyroid related antibodies are we testing?

For most patients, if we have clear hyperthyroidism and additional thyroid symptoms or signs, I only test TRab (thyrotropin receptor antibody). There are many types of TRabs. Some are stimulating-TSI (thyroid stimulating immunoglobulin); some are inhibitory.

I have also found that a great portion of Graves' disease patients have positive TPO antibodies (the diagnostic antibody for Hashimoto's thyroiditis). I even have patients who have had Hashimoto's hypothyroidism for over 40 years and then suddenly switched to hyperthyroidism (Graves' disease).

What are other causes of hyperthyroidism?

Hyperthyroidism, strictly speaking is when the thyroid synthesizes and releases too much thyroid hormone. However, in daily life, we refer to hyperthyroidism as a "high level of thyroid hormone in the blood stream" regardless of the source. Sometimes, we also refer hyperthyroidism as thyrotoxicosis.

Thyrotoxicosis associated with thyroid hormone overproduction:
- Graves' disease
- Toxic nodule or toxic multinodular disease
- Trophoblastic disease (too much hCG)
- Multiple pregnancy (too much hCG)
- TSHoma (pituitary tumor secreting too much thyroid stimulating hormone- TSH, very rare)
- Some form of excessive iodine
- Amiodarone induced thyrotoxicosis type I

Thyrotoxicosis without thyroid hormone overproduction (most with reduced production)
- Thyroiditis (viral or bacterial infection, autoimmune disease)
- Trauma
- Amiodarone induced thyrotoxicosis type II
- Other cytokine induced
- Extensive cancer invasion
- Iatrogenic (doctor prescribed too much thyroid hormone)
- Factitious (patients take too much without doctor's approval)

I had a patient who owned a health vitamin store. She took a supplement that she believed might help her energy. She got herself into very severe thyrotoxicosis which caused atrial fibrillation.

I also had a patient who was admitted to the hospital for "thyroid storm" and adamantly refused to admit taking anything. However, later I found out she had a history of radioactive iodine ablation treatment for Graves' disease. I also did thyroid ultrasound to confirm that she did not have thyroid gland anymore.

Do you use thyroid ultrasound and fine needle aspiration (FNA) as your diagnostic tools?

I use thyroid ultrasound more and more in a work up for hyperthyroidism. Thyroid ultrasound is easy to perform and very convenient. We can make the most differential diagnosis on the spot with thyroid ultrasound. It is harmless and saves patients money and time. Therefore, I use radioactive iodine uptake and scan less and less. Thyroid iodine uptake and scan used to be a major tool for diagnosis of overactive thyroid (hyperthyroidism/thyrotoxicosis).

I usually do not use fine needle aspiration (FNA) in diagnosing thyrotoxicosis unless metastatic cancer is suspected. This is an extremely rare condition. Occasionally, if a concurrent nodule is present in Graves' disease, I might consider FNA.

What is the cause of Graves' disease?

The exact cause for the production of these antibodies is not clear. However, it has been recognized as linked to the following:
- Your genes
  - Very often in the family. Doctors always ask your family history. The odds are very high that your

mother, aunt or someone else also has had Graves' disease.

- o Also, very common in a family with Hashimoto's hypothyroidism (another autoimmune thyroid disease).
- o The sibling recurrence rate for Graves' disease exceeds 10.0%.
- o If your monozygotic twin (identical) has Graves' disease, your chance of developing Graves' disease is 20-40%.
- o There are associations with a number of immune-related genes which have also been found with many other autoimmune diseases and presumably underpin the inherited susceptibility to autoimmunity.
- Virus infection. Graves' disease can be induced in animals by a certain viral infection.
- Female gender. The female to male ratio is close to 4:1.
- Stress. Stress has been implicated in developing Graves' disease/Hashimoto's thyroiditis.
- Smoking. Smoking is a risk factor for Graves' hyperthyroidism (relative risk approximately 2.0) and an even stronger risk factor for Graves' orbitopathy (Graves' eye disease).
- Pregnancy. Pregnancy leads to many changes in our immune system. A condition called postpartum thyroiditis is a variant of Hashimoto's thyroiditis. Graves' disease is also much more common than we thought after pregnancy.
- Radiation exposure. People working in the field of medical radiation have higher risk. People exposed to nuclear power plant accidents also have increased risk.
- Iodine and iodine-containing drugs such as amiodarone and computed tomography (CT) scan contrast media may precipitate Graves' disease, or a recurrence of Graves' disease, in a susceptible individual.

I do not have goiter (large thyroid). Do I have Graves' disease?

The majority of Graves' disease patients have a certain degree of goiter. I have patients who have Graves' disease but there is no goiter at all. Therefore, even if you have no goiter but have certain symptoms, signs and positive TSI, you have Graves' disease.

My thyroid function is always normal. Do I have Graves' disease?

There are reports of positive TSI, but with normal thyroid function. I have patients with Graves' eye disease, but normal thyroid function.

I also have patients with 40 years of hypothyroidism, and who suddenly switched to hyperthyroidism. I have patients with both positive TSI and TPO. Although the majority of Graves' disease patients have hyperthyroidism, you can have hypothyroidism or normal thyroid.

However, in the clinic setting, most doctors consider Graves' disease as a synonym for hyperthyroidism.

What kind of symptoms can I have if I have Graves' disease?

As stated above, most Graves' disease is presented as hyperthyroidism: anxiety, emotional lability, increased irritability, weakness, tremor, palpitations, heat intolerance, increased perspiration, and weight loss despite a normal or increased appetite.

Some patients with Graves' disease can also have eye disease or specific skin disease.

What is the manifestations in skin?

Hyperthyroidism brings changes in the skin from increased metabolism, blood flow and so on.

The following skin changes may occur:

- Warm, sweaty and smooth skin. When I greet a patient, I can sense the patient's thyroid status by shaking his or her hand.
- Pruritus (itching) and hives, which are occasionally found, primarily in patients with Graves' hyperthyroidism.
- Hyperpigmentation (increased skin darkness), which can occur in severe cases; very severe hyperthyroidism causes increased cortisol metabolism and increases the production of a pituitary hormone which increases skin color.
- Vitiligo (patchy skin color loss) and alopecia areata (patchy hair loss), which can occur in association with autoimmune disorders
- Thinning of the hair
- Graves' disease myxedema most present on legs-raised, hyperpigmented (increased skin color), violaceous, orange-peel-textured papules.

What are the manifestations in the eyes?

Stare and lid lag occur in all patients with hyperthyroidism. Patients might think they have proptosis (eyeball extrusion). Hyperthyroidism causes increased sympathetic nerve activity.

Graves' disease can cause Graves' eye disease (Ophthalmopathy). It is caused by inflammation of the extraocular muscles and orbital fat and connective tissue, which results in popping eyes-proptosis (exophthalmos), double vision (impairment of eye muscle function), and puffy eyes (periorbital and conjunctival edema). Smoking makes Graves' eye disease worse. Quitting smoking is important.

What are the manifestations in the hematologic system?

Anemia is common but, for most patients, this is not clinically significant. Patients with severe hyperthyroidism can have normochromic, normocytic anemia. Serum ferritin concentrations (correlated to blood iron level) may be increased.

Graves' hyperthyroidism is an autoimmune disease and may be associated with other autoimmune hematologic disorders such as immune thrombocytopenia (ITP) and pernicious anemia, and some patients have antineutrophil antibodies.

Hyperthyroidism may also increase the chance for blood clots since some of the clotting factors are increased.

Thymic enlargement. The exact cause is not known. I have a patient who I saw in the hospital after she had chest surgery for removing the enlarged thymus. it turned out that she had Graves' disease. Although not all thymic enlargement in Graves' disease need surgery, and treatment of Graves' disease with antithyroid medications, radioiodine, or thyroidectomy results in involution of thymic hyperplasia over 4 to 25 months, the chance for malignancy is increased. Repeat imaging three to four months after initiation of therapy is warranted to ensure regression.

What are the manifestations in the cardiovascular system?

Increased heart rate (sinus tachycardia) is very common. 10-20% can have atrial fibrillation, which is even more common in the elderly. Some also have premature beats or skipped beats. Patients may have symptoms of palpitation. 60% of atrial fibrillation patients reverted to normal after their hyperthyroidism was controlled. If not reverted to normal, then electroconversion is recommended. The recurrence rate is around 59% in two years. Blood thinner might need to be considered in some patients.

Systolic hypertension is also common in hyperthyroidism. Heart failure and severe cardiomyopathy can occur if hyperthyroidism is very severe and not controlled for a prolonged time.

What are the manifestations in the respiratory system?

The respiratory system is closely linked to the cardiovascular system and causes similar symptoms like fatigue, shortness of breath, and physical activity intolerance.

Hyperthyroidism increases the oxygen consumption and production of carbon dioxide which increases breath rate.

Hyperthyroidism also increases lung circulation and blood pressure which can also cause shortness of breath especially with exertion.

Hyperthyroidism can also cause respiratory muscle weakness.

Hyperthyroidism also exacerbates asthma.

The concurrent large goiter and thymus might compromise the breathing tube.

What are the manifestations in the digestive system?

Digestive system symptoms are another prominent presentation of hyperthyroidism. Most patients have increased appetite and increased gastrointestinal motility leading to loose stool, and increased frequency of defecation.

Abdominal pain and vomiting are rare presentation, but they can occur.

Increased liver function is very common in hyperthyroidism patients. Alkaline phosphatase is one very common parameter to be increased.

Can hyperthyroidism lead to weight gain?

Most patients have significant weight loss due to significantly increased metabolism. 10% of patients especially younger patients can have weight gain due to significantly increased appetite.

Weight gain also tends to occur in mild hyperthyroidism. These patients have significantly increased appetite, but the metabolism increase is not able to offset the increased eating.

I have a 35-year-old female who came to me for hyperthyroidism. She just cannot believe that she was continuing to gain weight while Dr. Google told her that with hyperthyroidism she should lose weight. After I explained to her why she gained weight, she said, "If my hyperthyroidism gets controlled, I expect to lose weight." The fact is that she might gain more weight. The reason is that the appetite is also part of habit. When you have the habit, you might continue to eat the amount you were eating. After controlling your thyroid function, your metabolism is reduced, and you might gain more weight.

I have a reduced appetite. Can I have hyperthyroidism?

Some have reduced appetite instead of increased appetite. This occurs more often in elderly patients. The reduced appetite and increased metabolism can lead to significant weight loss.

What are the manifestations in the urinary and reproductive systems?

Hyperthyroidism also increases urine production leading to polyuria (going to the bathroom more often) and nocturia (more often going to the bathroom at night).

Women with hyperthyroidism may have menstruation problems: too little, too heavy, too long, too short, or amenorrhea (no menstrual period). Fertility is reduced and the risk for abortion is significantly increased.

Men can have reduced libido (sex drive), reduced production of sperm and reduced fertility.

The total sex hormone is increased but the free, active hormone might be reduced. I have a 45-year-old man who was referred to me for increased total testosterone which was found during a reduced libido workup. He was found to have hyperthyroidism.

What are the manifestations in the nervous system?

Hyperthyroidism has very prominent manifestation in the nervous system and behavior changes. Most patients complain of anxiety, irritability and emotional lability.

Patients with hyperthyroidism can have lots agitation, restlessness, psychosis and even depression. I have seen a 22-year-old young girl admitted to the psych ward as maniac and found to have severe hyperthyroidism.

I also have seen an 85-year-old lady who was admitted to the psych ward for severe depression and was found to have hyperthyroidism. After the hyperthyroidism was resolved, her depression was controlled.

Insomnia is also common. Most patients have this complaint.

Severe hyperthyroidism can have cognitive impairments, particularly impaired concentration. If severe enough it can cause confusion, poor orientation and immediate recall, amnesia (forgetful), and constructional difficulties. I have a 20-year-old female college student. She was a straight "A" student but became a "C" student and was barely able to stay at college until she sought medical attention.

What are the manifestations in the musculoskeletal system?

The thyroid hormone is important for the muscles to work properly, but too much is not a good thing either. Muscle involvement in adults with hyperthyroidism is common. Patients may experience weakness, cramps, and myalgias. The serum creatine kinase (CK) is also frequently reduced.

Prolonged severe hyperthyroidism can cause myopathy which is manifested by severe muscle weakness.

The thyroid hormone has a severe effect on bones. It can cause calcium to go up (hypercalcemia) and bone loss. In elderly patients even, subclinical hyperthyroidism (mild form of hyperthyroidism) can cause osteoporosis (weak bone).

A few months ago, I was consulted in hospital for a 56-year-old university professor. When I walked into the room. I was surprised to see the patient crying. I asked what was going on. His wife stated that Dr. Google told him that there was an 80% chance he had cancer because his doctor just told him that he had elevated calcium but his parathyroid hormone (a hormone secreted by glands adjacent to thyroid regulating calcium) was normal. I told him that Dr. Google knows everything, but you need to ask the right question and you need to choose what to believe.

I spent the next 30 minutes explaining to him that the thyroid hormone actually increases bone metabolism and increases his calcium levels. He was treated with some intravenous fluids and started on antithyroid medication. He was discharged to home. I saw him again in the office a month later. His calcium was already normal, and his thyroid function was also so much better. He was still emotional but so much improved and calmer.

What is "thyroid storm"?

This simply means the ultimate severe kind of hyperthyroidism. It is so severe that you might die from this.

However, the diagnosis is not very clear cut. To different doctors, this can mean different things. I get calls from the ER or hospital ward often to be consulted for "thyroid storm". Instead, the patient just has hyperthyroidism.

How do you make the diagnosis of "thyroid storm"?

The good news is that I have not had any patient die because of "thyroid storm".

We actually have a score system to help doctors make the diagnosis. I usually just make the diagnosis on my own criteria. If my patients have any of the following, I would treat them as having "thyroid storm"; if two out of three, then I am certain the patient has "thyroid storm".

Anyone who has any of the following three symptoms:
- Fever >100 ° F, not due to obvious infection
- Mental status change including but not limited to agitation, psychosis, delirium, seizure, certainly coma.
- Compromised cardiac function, such as heart failure, atrial fibrillation with rapid heart rate, or heart rate >140.

Chapter 2. Understanding Thyroid Function Tests

How is thyroid function regulated?

Lots of important hormones are regulated by the hypothalamus and pituitary gland. The pituitary gland is a central command for many hormones. It is situated at the base of the brain behind the nose. The hypothalamus secretes a hormone called the thyroid releasing hormone (TRH). It then promotes the pituitary gland to release another hormone called the thyroid stimulating hormone (TSH). TSH then stimulates the thyroid to synthesize and release thyroxine (T4) and triiodothyronine (T3). The levels of T3 and T4 regulate TSH by feedback.

What do we see from a thyroid function test related to hyperthyroidism?

In hyperthyroidism, we usually see TSH suppressed below 0.1. All thyroid parameters, total T3, free T3, total T4 or free T4, are increased. Some thyroid antibodies like TPO or TSI can be normal or increased.

What is TSH?

TSH is a hormone secreted from the pituitary gland. It works like a thermostat. If the T3 and T4 levels are too low, then it turns up the TSH level. If the T3 and T4 levels are too high, then it shuts down the TSH level.

TSH regulates T4 and T3 release just like the thermostat regulates your house temperature. TSH is like the thermostat; T4, T3 are like the temperature at your house. If the temperature is too high, your thermostat will shut down; if the temperature is too low, your thermostat will start up. Same thing if your T4 and T3 are too high, TSH will decrease; if T4 and T3 are too low, TSH will increase. Certainly, the assumption is that your thermostat works properly; likewise, that your pituitary works properly.

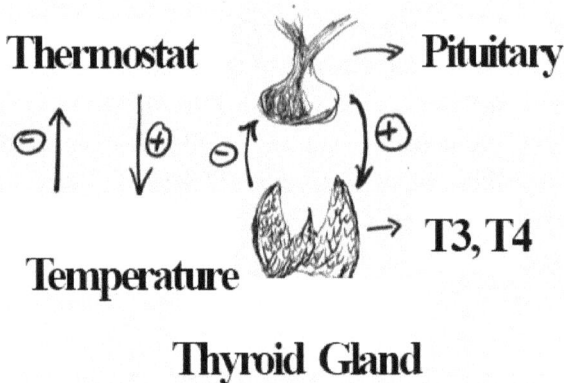

Fig. Illustration of the relationship of the pituitary hormone TSH and T3 and T4 just like a thermostat and the temperature. + indicating stimulating to cause T3 and T4 or temperature to increase; - indicating suppressing (feedback) to cause TSH to decrease or thermostat to shut down, and then T3 and T4, and temperature to decrease.

What is the normal value for TSH?

Different labs might give different normal values. Most labs give a normal value of 0.5-5 mIU/L.

At different ages, the normal value is slightly different. When we age the TSH value tends to increase slightly.
At each stage in pregnancy the TSH levels are different.

What non-thyroid conditions and drugs might affect TSH levels?

Some specialists and professional societies only recommend checking TSH levels which can miss the full picture since TSH can be affected by many conditions and medications. If you are very sick, your TSH can be low.

Many medications affect TSH values. The most common medications are steroids, dopamine agonists (bromocriptine, cabergoline), somatostatin (a hormone from the pituitary gland or another gland to suppress other hormone secretion), amphetamine, metformin (diabetes medication), amiodarone (heart medication), rexinoids, and opioids.

Is it true that taking too high a dose of biotin can affect TSH measurement?

Yes, biotin might affect the laboratory measurement but not its function.

How are T3 and T4 measured?

Under normal conditions, our thyroid secretes 80% T4 and 20% T3. Most circulating T3 are converted from T4 at peripheral tissues like the liver and kidney. For T4, in the blood, 99.98% are bound to proteins (thyroxine-binding globulin, transthyretin and albumin), while 99.80% of T3 is bound to proteins.

It is much easier and more accurate to measure the total hormone (protein bound+free). However, many conditions and medications can affect binding protein levels and then falsely affect the total hormone level. Therefore, I do not order the test very often. Unfortunately, the measurements for free hormones are not very accurate either.

What medications increase the total hormones but do not affect the thyroid's function?

- Estrogens
- Birth control pills
- Tamoxifen (for breast cancer)
- Mitotane
- Heroin
- 5-fluorouracil (5-FU, cancer medication)
- Methadone (addiction medication)

If you are told you have high thyroid hormone levels, you need to let your doctor know you are on these medications.

What medications decrease the total hormones but do not affect the thyroid's function?

Some medications can reduce the thyroid binding proteins and then the total hormone levels.

- Androgens (testosterone and similar hormones)
- Glucocorticoids (like prednisone)
- Lithium (can cause thyroid dysfunction)
- Phenytoin
- Propranolol (also inhibits the conversion from T4 to T3)
- Niacin (nicotinic acid)

What conditions increase thyroid hormone binding proteins and then increase the total hormones with normal thyroid function?

The following conditions might increase thyroid binding proteins and then increase the total hormone measurement:

- Pregnancy
- Acute /chronic liver disease (can go both ways)
- Adrenal insufficiency
- AIDS
- Familial dysalbuminemic hyperthyroxinemia is a type of hyperthyroxinemia associated with mutations in the human serum albumin gene.
- Familial hyperthyroxinemia due to increased thyroxine binding proteins.

What conditions decrease thyroid binding proteins and then reduce the total thyroid hormones with normal thyroid function?

The following conditions might reduce the thyroid binding proteins and cause the measurement of total hormones to be decreased:
- Critical illness (very sick)
- Sepsis (blood infection)
- Nephrotic syndrome (lots of protein lost from kidneys)
- Diabetic ketoacidosis (please read my diabetes book)
- Acute and chronic liver diseases (can go both ways)
- Chronic alcoholism
- Severe cirrhosis
- Severe malnutrition
- Acromegaly (enlarged body parts caused by a brain tumor)
- Cushing's syndrome or Cushing's disease (caused by an overabundance of steroids in the body)
- Familial thyroxine binding protein deficiency (gene mutation)

How do we measure Free T4 and Free T3?

The free unbound hormones are active, making more sense to measure them. However, the measurement is not so accurate due to the very low level of the free hormones. Again, only 0.02% of T4 are free hormone and 0.2% of T3 are free hormone.

There are two ways to measure Free T4 and Free T3:
- Estimation of Free T4 and Free T3 testing.
  - o Use two assays to check both total T3, T4, and binding proteins and then calculate the index.
  - o Use automated immunoassay-most commonly clinically used.
- Direct measurement. It is very technically demanding and not routinely performed. In very special rare situations, I might order it.

What medication can affect on automated immunoassay?

I have an abnormal thyroid function test, but my function is normal. Here are the common medications:
- Artificially increase Free T4
  - o Amiodarone (can truly increase T4 synthesis)
  - o Salicylate (greater than 2g/day)
  - o NSAIDS (nonsteroidal anti-inflammatory drugs)
  - o Biotin
  - o Heparin use
- Artificially decrease Free T4
  - o Seizure medication: phenytoin (Dilantin)
  - o Seizure medication: carbamazepine

What is TPO?

TPO represents thyroperoxidase, but when we are talking about it most people are thinking about the antibody of TPO. It is reported as a titer like 1: 120. When it is high, it usually means you have autoimmune thyroid disease.

Does TPO increase the risk of thyroid cancer?

It is reported that patients with autoimmune disease have higher risks for thyroid cancer. However, it is not concrete. Up until now, no professional societies suggest that you have to screen for thyroid cancer if you have an autoimmune thyroid disease like Hashimoto's thyroiditis.

There is no concrete data suggesting that thyroid nodules in a patient with increased TPO antibody have a higher risk for cancer.

Why is my TPO up and down?

The unstable nature of autoimmune disease is the cause of TPO increasing or decreasing, but also remember the testing is not often accurate. The lab sometimes changes assays which also make patients and doctors confused.

Therefore, please do not be too alarmed about TPO variations. I do not recommend checking them repeatedly.

Is there any treatment for increased TPO?

There is no concrete treatment. Some report that selenium might help. I recommend patients take 100 mcg of selenium (or selenomethionine 200 mcg) daily. In some patients TPO decreases with the selenium supplement.

Can I take too much selenium?

Yes, you can have too much. We call it selenosis. We can check your blood level. If your blood level is over 100 mcg/dl, you have too much selenium. If you have too much selenium in your blood, you might develop nail problems, hair loss, skin rash, fatigue and increased irritability. Some also reported garlic-smelling breath.

If more severe and long term, some cases of skin cancer, liver and kidney damage have been reported. I have also seen reports that an overdose of selenium is linked to developing diabetes.

What food do you recommend increasing my selenium level?

Healthy food like nuts and vegetables such as spinach have good levels of selenium.

What is thyroglobulin? Do I have a higher thyroid cancer risks if my value is high?

Thyroglobulin is secreted from normal thyroid follicular cells. It correlates to thyroid volume. The bigger the thyroid tissue, the higher the thyroglobulin. If the thyroid is inflamed, the value also increases. The high values do not increase the risk for thyroid cancer. Before surgery, I usually do not measure it.

When do you measure thyroglobulin?

If you are confirmed to having thyroid cancer (papillary or follicular) after surgery and/or radioiodine ablation, we measure it to monitor thyroid cancer recurrence.

What is calcitonin?

Calcitonin is a hormone secreted by parafollicular cells (c cells) in response to increased calcium. The thyroid cancer derived from c cells is called medullary thyroid cancer. It is found in 3-5% of all thyroid cancers.

Should I have calcitonin checked in evaluating my Graves' disease?

I do not recommend checking calcitonin routinely in evaluating Graves' thyroiditis unless you have been suspected to have medullary thyroid cancer by biopsy, by family or personal history of MEN2, familial medullary thyroid cancer, or pheochromocytoma.

I also check calcitonin on patients who have a biopsy showing follicular lesions including Hurthle cell lesion.

What is TRab?

TRab stands for TSH receptor antibody. It can be stimulating or inhibitory. If you have hyperthyroidism and you have positive TRab, we assume you have TSI (thyroid stimulating immunoglobulin). We say you have Graves' disease.

What is TSI?

Again, TSI is thyroid stimulating immunoglobulin. It is an autoimmune antibody. It can bind to the TSH receptor and work like TSH to stimulate thyroid cells to grow, to secret more thyroid function.

Do I need to be fasting before a thyroid function test?

No, you do not need to be fasting for a thyroid function test.

Should I take antithyroid medication on the day of testing?

If you are taking antithyroid medication, you should continue to take it as usual on the day of testing.

Should I take my thyroid supplement on the day of testing?

Your total and free T4 and T3 might increase slightly for the first four hours after you take your medication. Your TSH will not be changed.

I recommend my patients do whatever they usually do on the day of testing. No fasting and taking their medication as usual is recommended.

Some patients like to fast because they are accustomed to it. It is okay with me.

Chapter 3. Thyroid Ultrasound

What does a normal thyroid ultrasound look like?

The normal thyroid is very smooth, and consistency is very good. It looks whiter than muscle. Here is my own thyroid ultrasound.

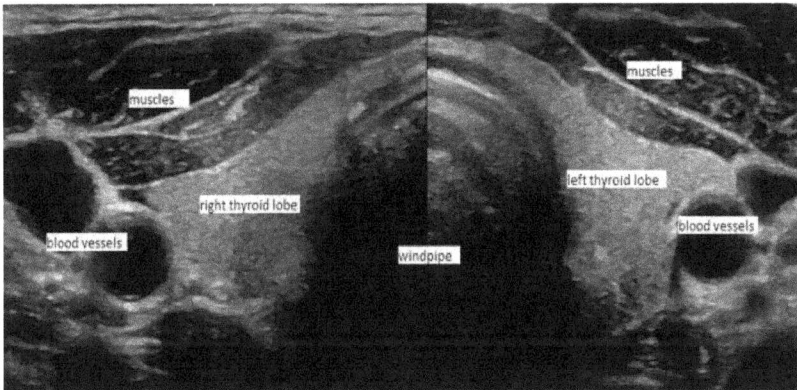

Figure: normal thyroid ultrasound

Should I have thyroid ultrasound in evaluating hyperthyroidism?

I recommend having at least one thyroid ultrasound. Thyroid ultrasound is becoming one of the most important tools in evaluating hyperthyroidism. There are many causes of hyperthyroidism. To name a few, we have Graves' disease, toxic nodules, and thyroiditis. In each situation, we can see the difference on the thyroid ultrasound.

These days, I rarely send my hyperthyroid patients for iodine uptake and scan. This test used to be the test for all hyperthyroidism patients.

Thyroid ultrasound actually saves a lot of money, time, and effort for my patients.

What are the typical features for Graves' disease on a thyroid ultrasound?

Graves' disease is an evolving condition. At the different stages, the ultrasound can show the differences. The heterogeneity and vascularity are the features. However, other conditions like Hashimoto's thyroiditis can also cause heterogeneity.

The thyroid can be enlarged or normal in size.

For subacute thyroiditis, we can see reduced vascularity.

For a toxic nodule or nodules, we can see the nodule or nodules. Sometimes we can see a high vascularity in the nodule or nodules. If this is the case, usually we have to order an iodine uptake and scan to differentiate from toxic nodule from warm or cold nodule (see my other book, <<*Thyroid Nodules*>>).

How do I prepare for a thyroid ultrasound exam?

You do not really need any preparation. I recommend wearing a low-cut shirt that makes the lower neck and thyroid area easily accessed.

I recommend not to wear neck jewelry while going to see a thyroid doctor. If you do, be prepared to take it off and store it properly.

Is there any harm to me?

We have not identified any harm or side effects for a thyroid ultrasound.

What is involved in a thyroid ultrasound exam?

We require that you lie flat on your back and, if possible, put a pillow under your shoulders to extend your neck.

Shunzhong Bao, MD

Chapter 4. Thyroid Radioactive Iodine Uptake and Scan

Why are we doing thyroid scintigraphy (nuclear testing - usually an iodine uptake and scan)?

Usually we do not need to have an iodine uptake and scan for making the diagnosis or managing hyperthyroidism.

I recommend having an iodine uptake and scan for the following situations:
- Patient has low TSH with a nodule or nodules.
- Patient has an overactive thyroid function test, but a thyroid ultrasound does not show significant increased blood flow (vascularity) and patient does not have neck pain especially when the ultrasound probe is being pressed on the neck.
- If patient has an overactive thyroid but no nodules and no TRab or TSI, we might refer them to have an iodine uptake and scan.

If you want to learn more about thyroid nodules, please read my other book *Thyroid Nodules, Questions From Real Patients*.

What is the best isotope for thyroid scintigraphy?

I-123 is the most common isotope used for thyroid scintigraphy. The dose usually given is 200-400 uCi.

Does the radioactive iodine uptake and scan hurt my thyroid?

The dose used for an iodine uptake and scan is very small. The effect on the thyroid is minimal and we only do it if you have an overactive thyroid.

However, we do want to make sure you are not pregnant if you are a female at reproductive age.

What precautions do I need to take after a radioactive iodine uptake and scan?

The dose is so small. Some experts even do not recommend to take any precautions, but I recommend washing your hands well after using the bathroom and do not handle other people's food and drinks for two days. Do not stay close to a pregnant woman or an infant for two or three days. Do not have sex for a week.

Do I need to stay away from certain foods before the test?

One week before the test, I recommend staying off:
- iodine vitamin supplements/iodized salt
- seaweed (kelp, etc), food containing agar, seafood (you might need to stay off longer)
- dairy products

Do you have a high iodine food list?

The following foods have high iodine content. If you are recommended to follow a low iodine diet, you should avoid this list.

See next page for the list (**also see the lower panel of the front cover**).

Food	Approximate Micrograms (mcg) per serving	Percent DV*
Seaweed, whole or sheet, 1 g	16 to 2,984	11% to 1,989%
Cod, baked, 3 ounces	99	66%
Yogurt, plain, low-fat, 1 cup	75	50%
Iodized salt, 1.5 g (approx. 1/4 teaspoon)	71	47%
Milk, reduced fat, 1 cup	56	37%
Fish sticks, 3 ounces	54	36%
Bread, white, enriched, 2 slices	45	30%
Fruit cocktail in heavy syrup, canned, 1/2 cup	42	28%
Shrimp, 3 ounces	35	23%
Ice cream, chocolate, 1/2 cup	30	20%
Macaroni, enriched, boiled, 1 cup	27	18%
Egg, 1 large	24	16%
Tuna, canned in oil, drained, 3 ounces	17	11%

31

*DV = Daily Value. DVs were developed by the U.S. Food and Drug Administration (FDA) to help consumers compare the nutrient contents of products within the context of a total diet. The DV for iodine is 150 mcg for adults and children aged 4 and older. However, the FDA does not require food labels to list iodine content unless a food has been fortified with this nutrient. Foods providing 20% or more of the DV are considered to be high sources of a nutrient.

Do I need to stay away from certain medications before the test?

You need to stop:
- Antithyroid medication for one week
- Levothyroxine three to four weeks
- Triiodothyronine (Cytomel, T3) one to two weeks
- Topical iodine two to three weeks
- Amiodarone up to six months
- Avoid iodine contrast mediums for CT scans for six weeks to six months prior. Currently, with the commonly used contrast you usually need to wait six weeks.

I am allergic to "iodine". What should I do?

You might be allergic to the iodine carriers but not the iodine itself. Therefore, you are not allergic to radioactive iodine which is a simple iodine salt. You should be okay having the test.

Do I need to be fasting before the test?

You are recommended to fast eight hours before the test. However, two hours after you take the pill you are allowed to eat. It is okay to drink some water.

What else should I prepare?

- I recommend wearing clothes which show your neck.

- Jewelry and other metallic accessories should be left at home if possible or removed prior to the exam because they may interfere with the procedure. You know the hospital is a public place. If you do not take good care of your jewelry, it can get easily lost.

How is the test done?

- The test is usually performed in a nuclear department in a hospital.
- After taking the pill, you will be asked to be back in four hours and also the next day for the thyroid scan.
- The scan usually only takes four to five minutes. During the process, you need to keep your neck still.

Should I have a PET scan for my hyperthyroidism?

No, you do not need a PET scan for diagnosis or managing hyperthyroidism. I have many patients who are referred to me because they found PET scan signals in their thyroid. The PET was performed for other reasons.

It is well known that Hashimoto's thyroiditis can result in a PET scan signal. However, I will do a thyroid ultrasound to make sure there is no more than Hashimoto's thyroiditis. So far, I have had no hyperthyroidism patients who were referred to me due to signals in the thyroid.

When should I have a thyroid CT scan or MRI?

If your thyroid is so big that your doctor cannot get the full picture of your thyroid, a CT or MRI might be ordered to look at the thyroid size and the extension in relationship to surrounding structures, especially with retrosternal extension (extension in the chest).

If a CT is ordered, usually non-contrast is recommended. High iodine in the contrast might cause worsening of hyperthyroidism. Therefore, if not urgent, I would recommend my patient to have a thyroid CT after their thyroid function has been controlled.

Chapter 5. How We Treat Hyperthyroidism: Medications

What are the main factors which affect the treatment decision?

The first and most important factor is the cause of hyperthyroidism. Besides Graves' disease, thyrotoxicosis (hyperthyroidism) can be caused by thyroiditis, taking too much thyroid hormone or taking a supplement containing thyroid hormone. Hyperthyroidism may also be induced by medication such as Amiodarone, or by taking too much iodine.

I have someone who was involved in an automobile accident and lacerated his thyroid. He developed thyrotoxicosis.

The second factor I pay more attention to is the severity. We certainly treat thyroid storm differently compared to regular hyperthyroidism. The thyroid function test is important, but the function does not correlate with symptoms very well.

The third factor is the age of the patient. Age is the number one predictor of cardiovascular disease. Patients who are younger than 40 years usually tolerate hyperthyroidism very well. I have a 20-year-old female whose thyroid function was off the chart, but she felt "fine" except for an increased appetite.

The fourth factor is the comorbidities. The most important comorbidity is cardiovascular disease. I usually take time to ask if the patient has a history of cardiovascular disease.

What is the goal of treating hyperthyroidism?

First, we want to control the symptoms. Second, we want to reduce thyroid hormone production and prevent worsening of your heart disease or prevent new issues with your heart. Third, we want to prevent recurrence.

Why do we use a "blood pressure medication" beta-blocker often in treating hyperthyroidism?

One of the most prominent cardiovascular presentations of hyperthyroidism is increased heart rate. Prolonged uncontrolled heart rate can cause heart failure, or possibly lead to atrial fibrillation.

What beta-blocker do you often use?

The most commonly used beta-blocker is propranolol. I usually prescribe 10-40 mg three times a day. It also blocks the conversion of T4 to T3. Again, T3 is the active hormone. This is also the beta-blocker which has the longest usage history in this setting.

What is the contraindication for propranolol?

I usually do not use it in patients with a history of severe asthma or active heart failure.

What can I take if I have a history of severe asthma or have current asthma attacks?

If you cannot take a beta-blocker due to asthma, I would try verapamil or diltiazem to control your heart rate. These are also blood pressure medications. They are called calcium channel blockers.

36

Can I take some beta-blocker once a day instead of three times a day?

Yes, you can take atenolol or metoprolol ER once a day. The goal is to reduce your heart rate down to below 80. If you have very mild hyperthyroidism and your heart rate is below 80, you do not need to take a beta-blocker.

When do you use an intravenous beta-blocker?

The emergency doctor sometimes uses esmolol 50-100 ug/kg/min for those patients who cannot take the beta-blocker orally or with "thyroid storm" patients to control their heart rate. Sometimes intravenous diltiazem is also used for atrial fibrillation with rapid heartbeat.

What are the anti-thyroid medications commonly used?

We have two antithyroid medications: methimazole (Tapazole) and propylthiouracil (PTU).

Which is better, methimazole or propylthiouracil (PTU)?

For most patients, methimazole (Tapazole) is the first choice since it is reported that propylthiouracil has more cases of liver failure.

When do you use propylthiouracil (PTU)?

I use propylthiouracil instead of methimazole in the following situations.
- Patient is allergic to methimazole.
- Pregnant woman in the first trimester.

- Some doctors like to use propylthiouracil when the patient is in a thyroid storm. Propylthiouracil also has the effect of reducing T4 to T3 conversion.

Of what side effects do I have to be aware when I am taking antithyroid medications (methimazole or propylthiouracil)?

All medications have side effects. The rate is not very high, which depends on how you count them. It was reported that 1-3% of patients develop side effects and cannot take the medication.

Like most medications, antithyroid medication can cause allergic reactions like rash or itching; gastrointestinal side effects like indigestion, nausea, vomiting, abdominal pain; skeletomuscular side effects like joint pain or muscle pain. Some patients also complain of headache, dizziness and loss of taste.

Can antithyroid medications cause liver failure?

Yes, both medications are reported to cause liver failure. Methimazole is much less, therefore we use methimazole more frequently. The good news is that the incidence is very rare. I have not had anyone who developed liver failure, but I have patients whose liver enzyme went up close to 1000. Fortunately, we caught it early and stopped the medication.

Therefore, when you are on antithyroid medication, you need to pay attention to your skin color and stool color. If you develop yellow skin, yellow eyes (jaundice), dark urine or pale stool (acholic stool), you need to stop the medication immediately and see your doctor at once. This is also the reason you need to follow up with your doctor if you are taking antithyroid medication.

My liver enzymes are elevated. Can I still take antithyroid medications?

As we discussed before, hyperthyroidism can cause your liver enzymes to go up. However, I would be very hesitant to give you antithyroid medication if your liver enzymes are five times above normal.

I saw a patient with severe hyperthyroidism. Her liver enzymes are six times sbove normal. I hesitated to start the medication and the second day the liver enzymes were over ten times above normal. Sometimes it can be very challenging.

My liver enzymes are elevated after taking antithyroid medication. Can I continue to take it?

Hyperthyroidism can cause elevated liver enzyme but usually not over three times higher than normal. Using propylthiouracil (PTU) much more frequently causes liver enzyme to increase, Up to 30% of PTU treated patients can have increased liver enzyme.

If the elevation is less than five-fold of up-normal, I would still use methimazole carefully while closely monitoring liver function. I would avoid any antithyroid medications especially PTU if the liver enzymes are greater than five-fold of up-normal.

I have a fatty liver. My liver enzymes has been gradually increasing. Can I still take antithyroid medications?

Fatty liver is the common reason why Americans have elevated liver enzymes and might gradually increase the level. Sometimes it can be over three times higher. If the liver enzyme is three times higher than normal for whatever reason, I would be very cautious in using antithyroid medication. If the liver enzyme is over five times higher than the upper limit of normal, I would avoid them if possible. If I have to use them, I would use methimazole and try a lower dose and closely monitor. I would check the liver function every week to make sure it is stable or improving.

I have a patient whose liver function had increased to over 500. I stopped methimazole and started other measures for thyroid. Her liver function gradually came down to normal in six weeks. I checked her liver function every week. It came down every time. Otherwise, I would have had to refer her to a gastroenterologist specialized in the liver. Fortunately, in my experience, this is not a common situation.

I saw my alkaline phosphatase is increasing on my patient portal. Is it dangerous?

Nowadays, patients are educated by "Dr. Google" and also learn all sorts of things from their patient portal. Anxiety also increases.

Alkaline phosphatase is also commonly increased in a fatty liver. Sometimes when severe hyperthyroidism has not been controlled, the bone fraction of alkaline phosphatase will increase. Certainly, if other liver enzymes like AST, ALT are severely increased (doubled or more than five times above normal), then you need to stop antithyroid medication and see your doctor immediately.

Do you have any patients who developed liver failure after taking antithyroid medications?

Fortunately, this is a very rare situation. Hepatocellular injury (defined as AST ALT > three times of upper normal limit) occurred in 2.7% of patients taking PTU and 0.4% of patients taking methimazole as reported. Liver failure (defined as requiring liver transplant) is much less. So far, there are a handful of cases reported in the world.

I do not have any patients who developed liver failure due to taking antithyroid medications. While it is recommended to closely monitor liver function while taking antithyroid medication, the occurrence is reported not reduced because of monitoring. It is believed to occur very acutely and rapidly.

What can I do to prevent liver failure?

You should avoid ingesting anything which might damage your liver, such as too much Tylenol or alcohol.

Also, when you are on antithyroid medication, you need to pay attention to your skin color and stool color. If you develop yellow skin, yellow eyes (jaundice), dark urine, pale stool (acholic stool), you need to stop the medication immediately and seek your doctor at once. This is also the reason you need to follow up with your doctor if you are taking antithyroid medication.

Can antithyroid medications cause bone marrow suppression?

Another very rare and potentially life-threatening side effect is bone marrow suppression. Bone marrow suppression can cause severely reduced white cells and therefore reduce your ability to fight infection. If you have febrile disease, you need to see your doctor promptly.

The effect of propylthiouracil is believed to not be dose dependent and the effect of methimazole is dose dependent. This is another reason we use methimazole more often.

I do not know anyone who died from this severe side effect. I have a 72-year-old female who came to me with severe hyperthyroidism symptoms. I started methimazole 20 mg three times a day. She was seen again in two weeks and was found to have white cells reduced by half. I stopped the medication and her white cells went back up to normal.

Can antithyroid medications cause other rare severe side effects?

Antithyroid medications especially PTU (propylthiouracil) was reported to cause vasculitis. Vasculitis can be a very severe condition which can cause fever, fatigue, headache, rash, joint pain and stroke-like symptoms. The longer you take these medications, the greater the chance you might develop these side effects.

Hypoglycemia (low sugar) was also reported from long-term use of antithyroid medications. It was believed to be related to the production of anti-insulin antibodies.

My neutrophils are low. Can I still take antithyroid medications?

It depends. Severe hyperthyroidism especially in African Americans can cause low neutrophils. If the number is below 1000 /mm^3, I would hesitate to start antithyroid medications. For patients below 1500/mm^3 but above 1000/mm^3, I would be cautious but might try and closely monitor.

What are the symptoms of low neutrophils?

Neutrophils are the white cells fighting infection. If neutrophils are low, you are prone to develop infection. Therefore, if you develop fever, chills, sore throat or an ulcer in your month, you need to see your doctor and check it out.

Do I have to take antithyroid medication forever?

It is a good question but not so easy to answer.

- If your hyperthyroidism is caused by subacute thyroiditis, you do not need to take antithyroid medications like methimazole or propylthiouracil.
- If your hyperthyroidism is caused by a toxic nodule, and you do not want to be treated with surgery or radioactive iodine, but antithyroid medication, then most likely you need to take it forever.
- If your hyperthyroidism is caused by Graves' disease, then you have a 50% chance to get into remission after two years of treatment. Unfortunately, I do not know the lifetime remission rate. In my experience, I have many patients who have recurrence at a much older age which causes more problems.

I have Graves' disease and I am taking antithyroid medication. Do you have any marker enabling you to predict recurrence?

As I discussed above, it is really difficult to know the life-time recurrence rate. It is believed that if your TRab (antibody) becomes negative from positive, then the chance to relapse is relatively low. It is reasonable to stop the medication at this time if the thyroid function is normal.

I took methimazole ten years ago without any problem. Now my hyperthyroidism came back. Does this mean I would not have a problem in taking antithyroid medication?

It is reported that severe side effects can occur in those patients who did not have any problem before. The risk is not clear to us, therefore, when we restart your antithyroid medication, we treat you as if you never took it before. We need to pay attention to side effects.

Can you tell me again why you do not like to keep patients on antithyroid medication forever?

I do not like to keep treating hyperthyroidism with antithyroid medication like methimazole and propylthiouracil forever for these reasons;

- Methimazole or propylthiouracil can have severe side effects.
- Due to the nature of Graves' disease, it is very common for the thyroid function to fluctuate. It is a common clinical scenario: the medication is reduced, and then the hyperthyroidism is worse; the medication is increased, and then the thyroid function is too low. Thyroid function plays such an important role for our body to function properly. Either way is not good.

When do you prefer to treat hyperthyroidism with antithyroid medication long term?

- Patient really dislikes the concept of surgery or radioactive iodine for whatever reason. I have a patient who believes that all parts of her body are given by God and we should not get rid of any part.
- Patient has high surgery risk and at the same time cannot follow the radiation precaution.
- Patient has very limited life expectancy, especially if they are living at a nursing home or other long-term care facility.
- Patient had previous neck surgery or neck radiation which formed severe scar tissue and at the same time, patient dose not want to have RAI.
- Patient has very mild disease and with negative or very low level of TRab or TSI.

I am okay taking antithyroid medication forever. Do you have any way to keep my thyroid function stable?

The unstable thyroid function most occurs in Graves' disease due to the unstable production of endogenous thyroid hormone.

I use the "Chinese way", suppress and replace, to treat unstable patients. I use a relatively high dose of antithyroid medication to completely suppress the endogenous thyroid hormone production and then use thyroid hormone replacement. This practice is very common in China; however, it is not common in America.

I always explain the strategy and rationale to patients and make sure they understand it. Otherwise, other doctors will be confused and stop one of the medications.

Do you use any other medications to reduce thyroid hormone?

Here are the other medications which we use to reduce thyroid hormone in some circumstances:

- SSKI
- Steroids
- Lithium
- Cholestyramine
- Rituximab
- Carnitine
- Chinese herbs

What is SSKI and when do you use it?

SSKI is a saturated solution of potassium iodide. When I was a resident, I remember it was used often by my attending physicians when preparing for thyroid surgery. It was believed that iodine may reduce the thyroid vascularity and reduce the intraoperative bleeding. I am a specialist. I do not use SSKI often. I like to control my thyroid patients well before sending them to surgery. The surgeons' technique might be better. There is a large study showing that there is no difference in giving or not giving iodine before surgery for Graves' disease.

Now I only use this medication when I think the patient has a "thyroid storm". It can reduce both T4 and T3 rather quickly. Usually I recommend five drops every six hours after starting methimazole or propylthiouracil at least one hour later for thyroid storm.

When do you use a steroid in treating hyperthyroidism?

I use a steroid in the following three situations:
- If I think the patient has a thyroid storm, I use 40 mg of prednisone daily if the patient can tolerate it. If not or in a true emergency, I give 300 mg of hydrocortisone once and then give 100 mg every six hours. Sometimes, dexamethasone is used 2-4 mg every 12 hours.
- If I think the patient has subacute thyroiditis. I usually give 20-40 mg of prednisone once daily until the pain is gone. I use less and less due to the side effects of high doses of steroids. I do not use them when the symptom of pain is not very severe or can be controlled by Tylenol or ibuprofen. I do not use it when you are young and do not have other cardiovascular conditions.
- I also use in patients who cannot use methimazole or propylthiouracil.

What is lithium and when do you use it?

Lithium is a mood stabilizer which has been used for bipolar, schizophrenia and other related conditions. It was found to have effects on thyroid function. It caused goiters, hypothyroidism and hyperthyroidism. It was reported that lithium was used in patients who could not tolerate methimazole or propylthiouracil.

I had to use it on one patient who had severe hyperthyroidism and developed severely increased liver enzymes and reduced white cells with the use of methimazole. However, at the same time, I started a steroid and cholestyramine. She was on 300 mg of lithium three times a day for two weeks. Eventually her thyroid function was reasonably controlled and followed by radioactive iodine treatment. She was successfully treated.

What is cholestyramine and when do you use it?

Cholestyramine is a bile acid sequestrant which is used for lowering cholesterol. It was found to also reduce the thyroid hormone reabsorption.

Cholestyramine is also being used off label for hyperthyroidism. I use it in the following situations;

- The hyperthyroidism is very severe, and I want to control it as soon as possible. You might think everyone with severe hyperthyroidism needs to get it controlled as soon as possible. This may be true, but for most patients I do not need to use this medication.
- Patients who cannot tolerate methimazole or propylthiouracil.
- Hyperthyroidism caused by subacute thyroiditis and it is desired to get control quickly either by patient or me.

I usually recommend 4 g two-four times a day. I usually give a jar with 378 g which is more affordable, and hopefully I do not have to give the second jar.

What are the potential side effects of cholestyramine?

It commonly causes stomach upset. Other side effects are abdominal pain, nausea, bloating, and constipation. Medication prescription information has a long list of side effects, so you might need to consult your pharmacist.

What is the interaction with other medications and how should I take it?

Cholestyramine affects a lots of medication absorption. I recommend that my patients take this medication one hour after taking other medications. It is a lot of work, but it is important. I have prescribed this medication for Amiodarone induced hyperthyroidism. If your Amiodarone has to be continued, this is very important. You have to take Cholestyramine at least one hour after taking Amiodarone, otherwise, the absorption of Amiodarone will be reduced.

In hyperthyroidism, we often use a beta-blocker like propranolol which can also be reduced in absorption by cholestyramine.

Therefore, I do not use this medication long term. Cholestyramine can cause deficiency of other essential vitamins and minerals.

What is Rituximab and why is it used for hyperthyroidism?

Rituximab is a monoclonal antibody used for treating severe rheumatoid arthritis and some lymphoma. It is believed that it attaches to the lymph cells and causes the cells to lyse. Graves' disease is an autoimmune disease. This is the reason Rituximab is used in treating

Graves' disease, however, I have never used this medication in treating Graves' disease due to its high cost and severe side effects (death).

What is carnitine and why is it used in hyperthyroidism?

Carnitine is a compound which works as a transporter shuttle long-chain fatty acid into mitochondria to be metabolized. It can be synthesized in the liver and many other tissues.

Carnitine inhibits both triiodothyronine (T3) and thyroxine (T4) entry into the cell nuclei. Thyroid hormone exerts its function through specific nuclear receptors.

What doses are recommended?

The specific dosage has not been well defined. I recommend the following:

- Acetyl-L-Carnitine: 2,500 mg per day.
- L-Carnitine L-Tartrate: 2,000–4,000 mg per day.
- Propionyl-L-Carnitine: 1,000 mg per day.

Can we monitor the effect of carnitine by measuring T3, T4 or TSH?

Unfortunately, carnitine is not inhibiting the synthesis of T4 or T3. Therefore, the level of T4 and T3 will not go down. TSH is not a good indicator either.

When do you recommend carnitine to patients?

I recommend carnitine for patients to try under the following circumstances:

- Patients with very severe hyperthyroidism and in conjunction with methimazole or propylthiouracil to control symptoms faster.
- Patients with intolerance to methimazole or propylthiouracil. I use carnitine with other medications like beta-blocker propranolol to control symptoms in preparing for radioactive iodine treatment. I never use it when preparing for surgery.
- Patients with subacute thyroiditis and wish to control symptoms faster.
- Patients took too much "thyroid supplement" causing severe hyperthyroidism symptoms.

Can I use some Chinese herbs to treat my hyperthyroidism?

I know there are many reports using Chinese medicine to treat hyperthyroidism. Unfortunately, I am not knowledgeable enough to make any recommendations. I have never used any.

Chapter 6. How We Treat Hyperthyroidism: Radioactive Iodine Ablation-RAI

What is radioactive iodine?

Iodine comes in different forms. The radioactive iodine we are talking about here is the form which can emit particles and can kill thyroid cells.

When do you recommend radioactive iodine for Graves' disease and some hyperthyroidism treatment?

I recommend radioactive iodine for hyperthyroidism treatment with the following conditions:

- All nonpregnant Graves' disease patients without significant thyroid eye disease (orbitopathy).
- If you have a "hot" nodule or nodules.
- If you do not want to have surgery or surgery is not recommended for you and you have a large goiter which produces symptoms like too much pressure, choking, or difficulty breathing.

If you have Graves' disease, would you take radioactive iodine ablation (RAI)?

I absolutely would take radioactive iodine. RAI has so many fewer complications compared to surgery. It is also so much easier. The only thing you need to do is to take the capsule and follow the precaution instructions. The advantages are no hospitalization, no anesthesia risk, no surgery risk, and no scar.

Which would you prefer-surgery or radioactive iodine treatment if you have a toxic thyroid nodule?

The decision is not so hard. I am in my 50s and my heart is healthy. I am not taking any medications right now. If I have a single toxic nodule or a toxic multinodular goiter, I would prefer to have the radioactive iodine treatment. Here are the reasons:

- Radioactive iodine involves no down time if you work by yourself. Otherwise, I recommend one week off from work.
- The risk is much lower. Although, theoretically it increases your chance to have cancer, the dose is very low, and the chance is very, very low.
- I can check my thyroid function regularly.
- I have a 50% chance of not having to take thyroid medication.

What are the specific conditions which make patients prefer RAI?

RAI is my default treatment for Graves' disease. If you have the following conditions, I would strongly recommend you have RAI:

- If you have severe heart or lung diseases which make you not a good candidate for surgery.
- If you have previous neck radiation (cause lots of scars).
- If you have previous neck surgery (cause lots of scars)

- If you are a singer, or other professional, your life is depending on your voice. I strongly recommend having RAI, since the risk for damaging your vocal cord nerve is zero.
- If you really dislike the idea of having a scar on your neck, you should take RAI.
- If you are prone to have keloid, you should strongly consider RAI.
- If you have a severe adverse reaction to antithyroid medications, I strongly recommend you have RAI. We have to use antithyroid medication before surgery. It is not necessary to use antithyroid medication before RAI.
- If you have an adverse reaction to anesthesia, you should take RAI.
- If you are elderly and frail, I strongly recommend RAI.

How long does the radioactive iodine (radioiodine) stay in your body?

Radioiodine stays in your body for only a short time. The radioiodine that does not go to thyroid tissue will be eliminated from your body during the first few days after treatment. It leaves your body primarily through your urine, but very small amounts can be found in your saliva, sweat, semen, and bowel movements.

I am allergic to seafood or to intravenous iodine contrast. Can I still use radioactive iodine?

Yes, you can. You might be allergic to the iodine carriers but not the iodine itself. Therefore, you are not allergic to radioactive iodine which is a simple iodine salt.

What is involved in radioactive iodine treatment?

The endocrinologist or nuclear medicine physician will give you a capsule of radioactive iodine (sometimes a liquid to drink) and you take it with a glass of water. That is it. Usually you only need to take it one time. A very small percentage of patients need a second treatment.

I have Graves' disease. What should I expect after radioactive treatment for thyroid function?

We expect to have a significant effect in 6-18 weeks. I usually see patients again in four to six weeks, so I can start thyroid hormone replacement promptly. I want to keep patients at low thyroid status as briefly as possible. Most hyperthyroidism patients have increased appetite, and this can become a habit. If thyroid function is too low, then the weight gain will be very significant. Certainly, some weight gain is normal, since severe hyperthyroidism can cause major weight loss.

I have hyperthyroidism. What should I expect after radioactive treatment?

- You might experience slight pain in the neck in the following days up to a few weeks.
- You might have cheek pain also (usually much less).
- You might experience neck swelling -with it becoming bigger in the following days or weeks, instead of becoming smaller.
- The symptoms of hyperthyroidism might get worse in the first one to two weeks after treatment.

I have a toxic nodule. What should I expect for my thyroid function after radioactive iodine treatment?

- After two years, about 90% of treatment success (thyroid function is under control) can be achieved. Usually the goiter is smaller.
- 28% (different rate with different reports) of patients develop hypothyroidism (low thyroid) at one year after radioactive treatment. Thyroid functions will need to be monitored long term.

How do I prepare for radioactive iodine treatment?

If you are taking an anti-thyroid medication like methimazole or propylthiouracil (PTU), you will need to stop taking it at least three days before. I usually ask my patients to stop five to seven days before the treatment if the thyroid function is suppressed too low.

- Follow a low iodine diet for one to two weeks if not urgent (see the front-cover lower panel for high iodine food). This includes avoiding:
    - iodized table salt (sea salt is ok if not iodized)
    - cough medicine
    - seafood (I usually ask patient to stay away longer)
    - vitamin supplements that contain iodine
    - dairy products contain some iodine, so you need to cut down on cheese, milk and milk products
    - eggs

You should also cut out any food colored pink with the additive E127 (more commonly used in Europe) such as:

- spam or salami
- tinned strawberries
- glacé cherries
- pink pastries or sweets (look on the labels for E127)

55

What should I do if I have been taking high iodine medications like Amiodarone?

Amiodarone has a very high level of iodine and can stay in your body up to ten years. I would recommend surgery if possible. However, I might still order an iodine uptake and scan to see if your thyroid can absorb any iodine. If there is some uptake, we still can treat with radioactive iodine although with a slightly higher dose. The failure rate might be higher. We might also be able to increase the thyroid absorption by giving you a recombinant TSH - Thyrogen.

What should I do if I have recently had a CT scan with a contrast agent?

Many agents have high levels of iodine. However, right now most agents can be eliminated from your body in two weeks if you have normal kidney function. Therefore, you can receive radioactive iodine treatment after a two week wait.

How long should I wait if I have used some topical iodine agent?

You need to wait at least two to three weeks.

When should I stop antithyroid medication?

For most patients, I do not pretreat with antithyroid medications like methimazole or propylthiouracil. However, I start antithyroid medication for the following situations:

- You are elderly and have severe hyperthyroidism, since after RAI, your thyroid level might go even higher.
- You have severe hyperthyroidism, but you have not yet decided to go ahead to have RAI.

I recommend stopping methimazole or propylthiouracil two to seven days before RAI treatment.

- If your thyroid function comes down to normal or is still high, I recommend stopping methimazole or propylthiouracil two to three days before RAI.
- If your thyroid function is suppressed too much, I recommend stopping four to seven days before RAI treatment. Usually it takes at least six days for thyroid function to rebound.

Should I stop beta-blockers?

No, you should not stop beta-blockers like propranolol or atenolol. These medications should be gradually tapered until your heart rate drops below 70.

Should I fast on the day of treatment?

You should fast overnight because doctors believe that iodine can be absorbed faster. If your treatment time is afternoon, I recommend fasting at least for four hours. However, it is okay if you have not been fasting.

What procedure is involved in this treatment?

If you are a woman at reproductive age, you will need a lab test to confirm that you are not pregnant.

Usually you will be instructed to be on low iodine for at least two weeks. On rare occasions, Thyrogen (recombinant TSH) is given for up to three days.

On the day of treatment, you are instructed to fast. It is okay to drink water. After reviewing the safety procedures, a capsule of radioactive iodine is given to you to take by a nuclear medicine doctor or your endocrinologist. You can eat after one to two hours. Again, if you have not been fasting, it is okay.

What are the side effects of the radioactive iodine treatment?

- Increased overactive thyroid: Radioactive iodine destroys your thyroid; thus, more thyroid hormones are released. Your hyperthyroidism symptoms might get worse initially before they are better.
- Metallic taste in the mouth: This can last for a few weeks.
- Nausea: This usually subsides one to two days after treatment. It is okay to take some nausea medications if needed. If you think you might vomit, you need to ask your doctor early for anti-nausea medications.
- Swollen salivary glands: This can last for a few weeks. This is caused by iodine absorbed by the salivary glands. Stimulating saliva flow a few days after treatment by sucking a lemon drop, for instance, is an effective remedy.
- Dry mouth: This can be a long-term annoying side effect. As recommended, drink plenty of water after the treatment and stimulate saliva flow by using lemon drops or lozenges. This is very important. I have a patient who developed annoying dry mouth and kept drinking water. He also developed hyponatremia (low sodium) which can be a severe condition.
- Treatment failure. There is a 10-20% treatment failure for Graves' disease. You might be treated again (go through another round) or you might choose to have surgery. I have a patient who had RAI treatment failure and he chose to have surgery. Afterwards, he was so happy because surgery is for sure and instant.
- Hypothyroidism: The majority of patients with Graves' disease will be hypothyroid if successful. I only have one person who had Graves' disease, was treated with RAI and a few years later her thyroid function is still normal, and she

does not need any thyroid hormone replacement. As discussed, up to 50% or more of patients with toxic thyroid nodule treated with radioactive iodine will develop hypothyroidism or low thyroid. The good news is that this is really easy to treat and if properly treated, there are no side effects.

- Cancer: This is a theoretical risk. The real risk is not known.

What can you do to minimize the worsening of an overactive thyroid after treatment?

Usually this is short-lived, and I do not worry about it. However, if you are elderly and your thyroid hormones are very high (above two to three times normal limits) with cardiovascular disease, I recommend pretreatment using an anti-thyroid medication like methimazole. This medication needs to be stopped at least three days before the radioactive iodine treatment.

You can also restart anti-thyroid medication three days after RAI.

Sometimes, I also use cholesterol medication Cholestyramine. This medication can be started one day after RAI.

I also recommend carnitine to some patients if they cannot tolerate antithyroid medications like methimazole, propylthiouracil or Cholestyramine.

When should I go to the ER?

Due to the destruction of the thyroid, swelling might develop. If you have tightening of the neck, difficulty breathing, or stridor following the administration of radioactive iodine, then you should go to the ER to be evaluated. I have never had any patient who has to go to the ER for that.

After RAI, the thyroid function might transiently increase. If you suspect that you might develop a thyroid storm, you need to go to the ER.

When do you restart anti-thyroid medication after radioactive iodine treatment?

I usually do not restart anti-thyroid medications after treatment. If your level is too high or you have a very severe cardiovascular disease, I would be worried about your thyroid hormone surging after the treatment. Then I would restart anti-thyroid medication three days after you take your radioactive iodine treatment. The thyroid function needs to be followed closely.

I also use Cholestyramine after treatment waiting one day after the radioactive iodine treatment.

Supplement carnitine can also be considered.

What can you do to minimize the chance of developing hypothyroidism (low thyroid)?

This can be tricky. For Graves' disease, I have hundreds being treated with RAI. So far, I only have one person who does not have to take thyroid hormone replacement.

For toxic nodules, your chance of not having to take thyroid hormone replacement is so much better. You have a 50% chance.

Some centers are giving a fixed dose while some centers calculate your dose based on your thyroid mass or nodule. We are sure that if we give you less radioactive iodine your chance of being cured (or controlling your thyroid function or shrinking your thyroid nodule or goiter) will be reduced. Usually the dose for treating Graves' disease is

10-20 mCi. For a toxic nodule, a toxic multinodular goiter, or goiter the dose ranges from 10-50 mCi.

When can I get pregnant after radioactive iodine treatment?

It will be verified by a lab test that you are not pregnant when you are treated. It is recommended not to get pregnant for at least six months. Ideally, do not get pregnant for 12 months especially if you plan to breastfeed. We also need some time to get your thyroid function to be stabilized.

Do I need to bank my sperm before receiving iodine treatment?

Usually the dose used for Graves' disease or a toxic thyroid nodule or a toxic multinodular goiter is relatively small. Although radioactive iodine can cause sperm counts to decrease, the fertility decrease is not clinically significant. It is not recommended for you to bank your sperm. However, if you know your sperm count is low to begin with, it is not a bad idea.

If you have metastatic thyroid cancer and are expected to have multiple rounds of radioactive iodine treatments, then banking your sperm is very reasonable.

When can I impregnate my wife after radioactive iodine treatment?

There is no specific recommendation, but this does not mean it is safe. Therefore, I recommend you wait for three months.

Shunzhong Bao, MD

When can I resume sexual activity?

I recommend no sex for two weeks. Condoms are strongly recommended especially for men treated with radioactive iodine.

After treatment can I take public transportation home?

I strongly discourage you from taking public transportation home to minimize your exposure to the public. If you are well enough, I recommend you drive home.

However, if you have to take public transportation home, sit as far away as possible from other people, especially from children or pregnant women.

Is there a time limit for taking public transportation?

Yes, again, I recommend you not take public transportation if possible on the first day. If you do, for the first day limit to two hours, then for the second day limit to three hours, the third day limit to four hours, and the fourth day limit to five hours. Airplane travel is strongly discouraged for a week after treatment.

When can I fly in an airplane and are there any precautions?

I recommend against air travel the first week, especially the first three days. Sometimes even after a week you still have radioactive iodine in your system and can trigger the alarm system in the airport. If you must travel, you might ask your treating physician to write a letter for you.

62

Do I need to obtain anything specific for the treatment?

Not really if you can take care of yourself. If you need other people to take care of you, or you have some specific conditions like a stool bag (colostomy) or a urine bag, then you need to get good gloves and wipes for your helper. Also obtain bags to store the materials you cannot flush down the toilet.

Should I stay in the hospital after treatment?

Usually you are released the same day.

Should I stay in a hotel to minimize contaminating my own house?

A hotel is a public house, so I do not recommend going to a hotel for that reason. However, due to your household situation, if you have small children or pregnant women at home and you are not able to stay six feet away (briefly passing by is okay), you might consider staying in a hotel. If you do, please take precautions as at your own home.

If you are treated for Graves' disease or toxic nodule or nodules, a three to four day stay at a hotel should be enough. If you have thyroid cancer and are treated with radioactive iodine, a week-long stay is more appropriate.

How long should I stay at home before going back to work?

If possible, you should stay at home for a week.

At night, how long should I sleep in a separate bedroom or beds at least six feet apart?

If you are treated for Graves' disease or toxic nodule:
- Away from adults for at least a week.
- Away from infants, children younger than 16, or pregnant women for at least two weeks.

If you are treated for thyroid cancer:
- Away from adults for at least 11-14 days.
- Away from infants, children younger than 16, or pregnant women for at least three to four weeks.

During the daytime, how long should I stay away from infants, children younger than 16, or pregnant women?

I usually recommend at least a week.

What else can I do to minimize contamination?

For the first week, it is recommended to:
- Not prepare food for other people
- Not share utensils with other people
- Not share towels with other people
- Wash hands very well after using the bathroom
- For men, sit down to urinate
- Wash your towels, bed linens, underwear, and any clothing stained with urine or sweat separately
- Make arrangements for others to provide childcare for infants and very young children

Is there anything I can do to minimize radiation to myself?

- Discuss with your doctor about avoiding excessive doses.

- Fast before the treatment but you need to drink water to keep yourself well hydrated. Fasting makes the radioactive iodine be absorbed faster and get through your gastrointestinal system faster.
- Do not eat immediately after taking the radioactive iodine. Wait at least one or two hours afterwards.
- Drink plenty of water and urinate frequently.

- If you are being treated for thyroid cancer and have been taken off thyroid medication to increase your TSH, you should not drink water excessively because it might cause severe low sodium which can be life-threatening. You still need to keep yourself well hydrated. This can be tricky. For most people especially a younger person, you should be okay. For the elderly and especially if you are taking some diuretics, you should not drink too much water.
- Try some sour lozenges to increase production of saliva to reduce the radiation to your salivary glands.
- If you are treated for thyroid cancer, you can resume your thyroid medication the next day.

When should I come back to see my doctor after RAI?

I see my patients in four to six weeks after treatment and then every four to eight weeks until the thyroid function has stabilized. Then I might see my patient every six to twelve months depending on the stability and any complaints. If you have lots of worries about weight gain, you should see your doctor often. If you gain significant weight or have symptoms of hypothyroidism (opposite of hyperthyroidism, are depressed, sleepy, have dry skin, dry hair, constipation, etc), you should consult your doctor as soon ass possible.

I know someone who gained a lot of weight after RAI. Is there anything I can do to prevent that?

This is actually very complex. As we discussed before, hyperthyroidism stimulates appetite and metabolism. When the metabolism is so high, even when you eat more you might still lose weight. The majority of hyperthyroidism patients experience various degrees of weight loss. 10% of patients even gain weight while contending with hyperthyroidism.

Our appetite and our way of eating can become habitual. Lots of patients take a few months of hyperthyroidism and then see their doctors and get diagnosed. Then it takes time to be referred to an Endocrinologist. The habit of eating is already formed.

When the RAI begins to have effect on the thyroid function, it initially might have an uptick bump but then gradually comes down. The metabolism is coming down, but because of the habit of eating as before, while the metabolism is coming down significantly, you can expect to regain some weight.

What you can do is to be vigilant and curb your diet while your hyperthyroidism is being controlled.

Another thing you need to pay attention to is keeping your doctor appointments. I have a patient who did not listen to what I said. She was supposed to come back to see me in six weeks, but for some reason she did not come until six months. By that time, she had gained 50 lbs and had severe hypothyroidism. She felt depressed and had all the symptoms and signs of severe hypothyroidism. Long-term hypothyroidism can be dangerous and may cause dementia or heart failure.

As a doctor, what can you do to prevent weight gain?

- I always warn my patients about the weight gain. The more you pay attention to it, the better you will be.
- If needed, I provide diet and exercise recommendations.
- I always closely monitor their thyroid function and start thyroid hormone replacement early or as soon as possible. I usually do not wait until the thyroid function is below normal. I start to supplement as soon as I see the function trending down. Sometimes I use thyroid ultrasound to monitor the effectiveness of RAI.

When do you declare the RAI treatment a failure?

We define the success of RAI treatment based on the controlling of hyperthyroidism without using any medication to lower or block the thyroid function, especially without using methimazole or propylthiouracil.

For Graves' disease treated with RAI, the thyroid function begins to reduce starting after four to six weeks. 40% will have hypothyroidism in eight weeks; 80% will have hypothyroidism in 16 weeks (four months). If your thyroid is not controlled after four months, most likely you have RAI treatment failure. Officially you need to wait for six months. However, I do not wait that long before retreating with RAI or recommending surgery.

Shunzhong Bao, MD

Chapter 7. How We Treat Hyperthyroidism: Surgery

When would you prefer surgery over the radioactive iodine procedure?

I would recommend surgery over radioactive iodine for the following scenarios:

- You have moderate or severe Graves' eye disease (orbitopathy), since RAI might make your eye disease worse.
- You have other heart conditions and want to get hyperthyroidism under control as soon as possible, and you can tolerate surgery. If your cardiologist is not okay with the surgery, we can still recommend medication and then radioactive iodine treatment if necessary.
- Your living conditions do not allow you to follow up with your physician frequently.
- Your goiter or nodule is so big that it affects your breathing or swallowing.
- You might also have thyroid cancer, even if you just have a benign nodule or nodules.
- If you are pregnant or breastfeeding or have pregnant women or small children at home, you might consider surgery.
- You are planning to get pregnant in the next six months.
- You have been or are taking medications like Amiodarone.
- You also have parathyroid adenoma (you are going to have neck surgery anyway).

What is involved with thyroid surgery?

You usually will be admitted to the hospital on the day of surgery. You will have general anesthesia which means you will have a breathing tube while undergoing surgery.

A small cut (depending on the type of surgery) will be made at the base of your neck along the skin crease to minimize showing the scar.

The surgery itself usually lasts one to two hours.

The surgical procedure involves proximity to large blood vessels, nerves for voice (recurrent laryngeal nerves as well as the external branches of the superior laryngeal nerve), and also parathyroid (governing your calcium balance).

What questions should I ask my surgeon?

We usually refer you to a surgeon we think is very good, but the relationship needs to be personal. At the consultation, you need to ask questions and see if you feel comfortable letting the surgeon do the job.
- How many thyroid surgeries do you perform annually?
  - Some research reports that surgeons who do over 25 cases per year have fewer complications.
- Do you follow current thyroid surgery guidelines? If not, why not?
  - Guidelines are very important in deciding how to treat, but the surgeon also needs to understand your specific condition.
- Do I really need surgery? What are the alternatives? Advantages and disadvantages?
- You are referred to have surgery. This does not mean you have to have surgery.
- What are the possible complications?
- What are your chances of complications?

- o Thyroid surgery can have complications. See below. While asking these questions, you might be able to sense how confident his or her responses are.
- o I do not like the answer "I do not know". I believe when doing anything, if you track what you do, you do better. When a surgeon does not know what his or her complication rate is, then he or she might not focus on improving himself or herself.
- If you have worries for a particular complication such as loss of voice, ask for the last time this happened to his or her patient. What was the possible reason?
- Is there anything the surgeon can do to reduce the risk?
- What is his or her plan? Based on your condition, what kind of surgery is he or she planning to do?
  - o Depending on your current diagnosis, is the surgeon planning to remove just the nodule? Lobectomy? Near total thyroidectomy? Complete total thyroidectomy? Need to remove lymph nodes?
- If you worry about the scar, ask to see if you can get a plastic surgeon for the cut and closing. What product does he or she recommend for your healing? Anything else you need to do to reduce the scar formation? If you tend to form large "ugly scares" (keloid), tell them now to see if they can do anything.

What are the potential complications for thyroid surgery?

Surgery can have complications, but currently surgeons are better, too. However, the complication rate is absolutely surgeon dependent. I only refer to surgeons who have lots of experience and I communicate my perspective for the particular patient to them. Following are the complications which might happen:

- Bleeding, especially for patients with bleeding disorders. This can be very dangerous and life threatening.
- Neck swelling - seroma, causing bulging but no significant pressure symptoms.

- Infection is rare, and I have not seen one.
- Nerve damage causing hoarseness. If severe enough, it can cause breathing difficulties.
- Numbness and tingling caused by damage to the parathyroid gland which is very important in maintaining blood calcium level. If calcium is very low and not corrected, it can not only cause spasms, but it can also cause irregular heartbeats and be life threatening.
- The surgeon will also discuss other complications with you such as anesthesia reactions which can even cause death.

What is my down time following surgery?

Thyroid surgery in most centers involves an overnight stay. Most patients have told me that they did not need any pain medication.

It is a good idea to stay home for one week.

What are my restrictions after surgery?

Until the first follow-up appointment after surgery, you should restrain from:
- Talking too much, yelling, or singing.
- Bending down or doing any strenuous activity.
- Lifting any heavy objects.
- Driving if you do not have full motion of your neck.

What do I need to pay attention to?

You need to pay attention to the following. If any of these occur, do not hesitate to call your surgeon or go to the ER.
- If you have fever, or unusual pain, you might have an infection.
- If your neck swells, especially with pressure.
- If you have choking, especially with too much pressure and especially difficulty breathing.

- If you have numbness and tingling, you can try taking more calcium. If not relieved, call your doctor or go to the ER.

I have a scratchy voice. Does it mean my vocal cord nerve is damaged?

No. You had a breathing tube going between your vocal cords and these might have a small degree of trauma which causes your scratchy voice. It can take up to one or two weeks to heal.

Due to the surgical procedure, the edema, swelling and temporarily compromised blood flow might affect nerve or muscle movement that make the voice. This can cause some difficulty in speaking. This should improve in a few weeks.

This is one of the reasons I recommend not talking too much, yelling, or singing.

How do I know my voice nerves have been damaged?

If you have difficulty breathing while talking and it is very difficult to speak, then most likely your voice nerves have been compromised.

Do not panic. If you panic, it will make your breathing even more difficult. Your surgeon will help you to find the right physician or speech therapist to help you.

Will I have an ugly scar on my neck?

It actually will depend on your own skin's ability to heal. Some patients that tend to have keloids most likely will have trouble. Most patients will not have an ugly scar. The surgeon will make as small an incision as possible along the skin crease to minimize the scar showing.

If this is very important for you, you need to talk to your surgeon about it. Together you can decide if you need a plastic surgeon to assist for the cut and close.

There is a report of an alternative route from the axilla or mouth to make the cut. I do not know any surgeon who does that in my area.

Can I do anything to reduce the scar?

Most people heal well. A cut in the neck usually heals nicely.

I have patients who use silicone gel, or hydrogel and apply it to the incision daily for some extended time (three months or more). I also have patients who use the Mederma Advanced Scar Gel and believe it helps.

You should also protect the scar from sunlight for the first three months. Patients have reported that using sunscreen is very helpful.

When you talk to your surgeon, you can ask for more suggestions.

Can we reduce the chance of any complications?

- I refer my patients to a surgeon with a good track record. Different surgeons create different outcomes.
- I will check your vitamin D and calcium levels before surgery. I will start vitamin D supplements before sending you to have surgery.
- Closely monitor your calcium after surgery.
- Have an ENT doctor check your vocal cord before surgery if you have concerns for your voice.

Do I always need calcium tablets after surgery?

No, this depends on the damage to the parathyroid glands. We have at least four of them, two on each side. If you just have a lobectomy (half of your thyroid removed), you do not need extra calcium since we know at least the other two are working.

When you have a total thyroidectomy, the surgeon may not be sure if he or she can identify the parathyroid glands and preserve them. We can check your PTH the second morning. If they are low, then you need calcium, vitamin D or active vitamin D calcitriol depending on your calcium level. However, before surgery, I always check my patient's vitamin D to make sure they have adequate vitamin D.

When can I get pregnant after thyroid surgery?

I recommend getting your thyroid hormone optimized before becoming pregnant. Thyroid hormone is very important for pregnancy. It is not just for getting pregnant and a healthy pregnancy. It is also crucial for fetal brain development.
Make sure to communicate with your endocrinologist before you become pregnant.

Will thyroid surgery affect my sex life?

You can resume sexual activity as soon as you feel like it. Thyroid surgery itself does not affect your sex life long term, but if you do not have your thyroid hormone balanced, then your sex life can be affected. The thyroid hormone affects every cell, every tissue, every organ in our body. Therefore, after thyroid surgery, you need to follow up with your endocrinologist or internist to make sure your thyroid hormone is balanced.

Can I have a partial thyroidectomy and then not have to take thyroid hormone replacement?

If you have Graves' disease, usually you will have subtotal thyroidectomy where most thyroid tissue is removed, but not trying to get everything. However, you will need thyroid hormone replacement.

If you have a toxic nodule, potentially you can have a lobectomy or part of the thyroid removed depending on the location of the nodule. You might not need thyroid hormone replacement.

I heard that some centers use alcohol injection to treat thyroid nodules. What do you think?

At some centers, alcohol is being used to treat benign and simple cystic nodules. I have patients who had the treatment and said the procedure caused very significant pain. Also, the post treatment thyroid ultrasound will not look good which might confuse the treating physician afterwards.

However, if you have access to an experienced physician it should be a safe procedure especially if you have other comorbidities which increase your risk for surgery. This can be a good option for you.

Do I have any other non-surgical options for a toxic thyroid nodule or nodules?

For non-cancerous nodules, if the patient does not want to have surgery or surgery is not desirable, some centers offer laser ablation, cryoablation, and radiofrequency ablation to remove the benign nodule. I recommend using radioactive iodine. Please see Chapter 6.

Shunzhong Bao, MD

Chapter 8. Special Situations: Subclinical Hyperthyroidism; Hyperthyroidism with Pregnancy

What is subclinical hyperthyroidism?

Subclinical hyperthyroidism is defined as normal serum free thyroxine (T4) and triiodothyronine (T3) concentrations in the presence of a subnormal thyroid-stimulating hormone (TSH) (<0.5 mU/L).

I do not have any symptoms. Can I have subclinical hyperthyroidism?

The definition of subclinical hyperthyroidism is biochemical. It is not related to clinical symptoms since the clinical symptoms are very nonspecific.

How common is subclinical hyperthyroidism?

The prevalence of subclinical hyperthyroidism in the community varies between 0.7 and 12.4 percent.

What are the causes of subclinical hyperthyroidism?

Any causes of overt hyperthyroidism can also cause subclinical hyperthyroidism.

What is the most common cause of subclinical hyperthyroidism?

In America, as many as 10 million patients are taking thyroid medications. The exact number of patients who have subclinical hyperthyroidism is not clear but many of them have subclinical hyperthyroidism. In my experiences, the chance of having subclinical hyperthyroidism is much higher if the patient is taking desiccated thyroid products like Armour thyroid. Recently I saw an elderly man who was on levothyroxine. He has lots of anxiety and insomnia. His TSH was very low but with normal FT3 and FT4. I reduced his dose. Some of his symptoms went away.

There are many cases of subclinical hyperthyroidism which are caused by all sorts of supplements for "energy" and "weight loss".

What are other causes of subclinical hyperthyroidism?

Other common causes are:
- Autonomously functioning thyroid adenomas and multinodular goiters
- Certain stage of Graves' disease (very early stage, late stage, or under treatment)
- Certain stage of thyroiditis
- Other medications like Amiodarone, high dose of iodine, iodine content imaging contrast
- Other medications like steroids
- Certain stage of pregnancy

Why are the measurement of TSH, FT3 and FT4 inconsistent?

Some of my patients are really smart. They ask really intelligent questions. TSH, FT3 and FT4 are all measuring the thyroid function. They should be consistent, but why do we have the situation that TSH is low but FT3 and FT4 are normal?

I think this situation can be explained from the following two aspects:
- First, TSH is secreted by the pituitary gland. It is like an internal monitor which is much more sensitive than we can measure FT3 and FT4. In other words, your body knows the thyroid function changes before we can measure the difference between normal and high FT3 and FT4.
- Second, the normal lab value is derived from a range which would cover 95% of the referred as "normal people".

What are the symptoms of subclinical hyperthyroidism?

Most subclinical hyperthyroidism does not have any symptoms at all. Some patients do have symptoms of overt hyperthyroidism like anxiety, insomnia, changes of appetite, or changes in weight. Lots of patients with subclinical hyperthyroidism have weight gain instead of weight loss due to the increase of appetite.

Subclinical hyperthyroidism has also been associated with atrial fibrillation which increases the risk for stroke and low bone mineral density which increases the risk of fracture.

Is it true that subclinical hyperthyroidism increases mortality?

There are a few population studies reported that show subclinical hyperthyroidism increases slightly both the all-cause mortality and cardiovascular mortality.

Is it true that subclinical hyperthyroidism increases dementia?

Subclinical hyperthyroidism also increases the rate of dementia.

How do you make the diagnosis of subclinical hyperthyroidism?

The diagnosis of subclinical hyperthyroidism is based on biochemical testing. It disregards the symptoms and signs.

If you have low TSH and normal FT3 and FT4 then you have subclinical hyperthyroidism. Certainly, we still need to make the differential diagnosis.

What else do you consider in deciding treating or not treating subclinical hyperthyroidism?

There are many causes of subclinical hyperthyroidism. I try to figure out which is the cause for a particular patient and then decide how to treat or not.

I also make sure to differentiate other conditions which might have similar biochemical readings.
- Central hypothyroidism. Patients have low TSH and low FT3 and FT4 but sometimes the FT3 and FT4 can be close to normal. This is very important since one is overactive thyroid and the other is underactive thyroid. The treatment is opposite.

- Nonthyroidal illness. If a patient is very sick, TSH is suppressed and most of the time FT3 is low. However, sometimes FT3 and FT4 are still in the normal range. This is also very important to recognize. Lots of sick patients also have other conditions like atrial fibrillation, which might lead some inexperienced physician to start antithyroid medication, but in reality, these patients have low thyroid to start with, and antithyroid medication might cause harm to them.
- A certain stage of thyroiditis can have a similar picture. In this situation, the thyroid is damaged and leaks out a low level of thyroid hormone. It is not really over-producing. If antithyroid medication is used, then it might cause harm.
- Normal is just a lab value to cover 95% of normal people. In other words, in any period of time, 2.5% of normal people will have a low number and 2.5% of normal people will have a high number. They are just a number which does not mean they really have something wrong.
- A different ethnicity might have a different "normal value", however, right now they are reported the same. It is reported that African Americans have a lower normal TSH, however it is not reported on the lab report. To make things more complicated, how about those people with mixed ethnicity? No one really knows their normal value.
- Taking a high dose of biotin can cause the erroneous low TSH value.

What tests might you order?

For most patients, I might not do further testing. I make the differentiation from patient history and after reviewing their medications.

The most common test I do is a thyroid ultrasound which can tell me a lot about the thyroid.

We sometimes have to do the tests for hyperthyroidism to make the differential diagnosis (see previous chapter).

Who will you treat?

I consider the following factors:
- Even for subclinical hyperthyroidism, I want to make sure that the patient truly has hyperthyroidism.
- I am more inclined to treat if the patient's age is greater than 60.
- If the patient has some sort of symptoms like anxiety, weight loss, insomnia, sweating, and so on.
- If the patient has some sort of cardiovascular disease, like coronary artery disease, atrial fibrillation, heart failure, tachycardia, angina, etc.
- If the patient has osteoporosis, or with worsening bone mineral density.

How do you treat subclinical hyperthyroidism?

For the patients I decide to treat I would treat like overt hyperthyroidism patients. However, these patients might be elderly and have very mild symptoms, so I might try a very low dose of antithyroid medication. I also recommend RAI more often if needed. Surgery is usually less recommended.

For those patients overdosing on thyroid medications, we certainly recommend adjusting the dosage and further education about how to take thyroid medication, so they can be more stable.

Section: Hyperthyroidism and Pregnancy

What are the physiological changes during pregnancy?

Thyroid function is crucial to becoming pregnant and to maintaining pregnancy. There are many changes.

First, the pregnancy hormone chorionic gonadotropin (hCG) has a similar structure of TSH, which stimulates thyroid cells to produce more thyroid hormone. 1 IU of hCG is equivalent to 0.0013 IU of TSH. In an early pregnancy, or with multiple pregnancies or hyperemesis gravidarum, the hCG can be very high and cause subclinical hyperthyroidism or even overt hyperthyroidism.

Second, pregnancy causes serum thyroxine-binding globulin (TBG) to increase, and so the total T3 and T4 are increased. Therefore, when we check the thyroid hormones during pregnancy, we do not only check the total T3 or T4, because they are very high.

Third, pregnancy is a status of immunosuppression. Some Graves' disease patients have remission. I have a patient with Graves' who goes into remission every pregnancy. I saw a case report that the circulating thyroid-stimulating immunoglobulin (TSI) gets into the fetus and acts on the fetus' thyroid to cause hyperthyroidism in the fetus. When I was a fellow, I was really worried about this situation. However, nature has been able to take care of it. The production of TSI is apparently suppressed during pregnancy.

Fourth, pregnancy also has been associated with thyroiditis. Postpartum hypothyroidism is a phenomenon after pregnancy.

How is thyroid function evaluated during pregnancy?

Sometimes it can be very challenging to assess thyroid function during pregnancy. High hCG stimulates thyroid to grow and take more iodine and to make more thyroid hormones. Partly I think this is to help your fetus to develop. There are lots of studies on the hCG on the thyroid gland. Some report suggested that 50,000 IU of hCG is roughly equivalent to 35-65 IU of TSH. I saw a 19-year-old patient with a twin pregnancy. She had hCG over 220,000. She had severe overt hyperthyroidism. Again, normal nonpregnant TSH is in the range of 0.5-5. During pregnancy, different stages have different normal value. For T3, and T4, most likely we check FT3 and FT4. Sometimes, we also estimate the normal value of total T3 and T4. We consider the total T3 or total T4 to be high if the values are higher than 1.5 times above nonpregnant normal value.

Second, the pregnancy status is the status of immunosuppression. Graves' disease is an autoimmune disease and the severity of Graves' disease is significantly relieved due to the immunosuppression. I had a patient with moderate Graves' disease and every time she got pregnant, her thyroid function became close to normal and I did not need to give any medication. Therefore, you have to be very careful if you are taking antithyroid medication and get pregnant. Your antithyroid medication might have to be reduced and stopped. After delivery, we had to restart medication. The TSI might be negative. I repeat TSI postpartum if needed.

Third, due to the immunity change, patients have an increased risk of developing thyroiditis postpartum. Thyroid function needs to be repeated after pregnancy.

What are the causes of hyperthyroidism during pregnancy?

Any cause which can cause nonpregnant women to have hyperthyroidism can cause pregnant women to have hyperthyroidism.

Here are a few pregnancy specifics:

- Graves' disease might be subsided. When I was a fellow, I read a case report about a mother with Graves' disease and the mother's antibodies got into the fetus and caused the fetus to have hyperthyroidism. I was really worried about that Graves' diseased mother. The reality is that most Graves' diseased mothers will do well since nature has already taken care of it. During pregnancy, Graves' disease subsides.
- Some patients with multiple pregnancies have severely elevated hCG which can cause hyperthyroidism and might need treatment.
- Some patients with hyperemesis gravidarum who have severely elevated hCG which can cause hyperthyroidism and might need treatment.
- Some patients with trophoblastic hyperthyroidism — Hyperthyroidism can also occur with gestational trophoblastic disease. If a hydatidiform mole (molar pregnancy) is benign and it may give rise to choriocarcinoma. Both are associated with extremely high serum hCG concentrations and abnormal hCG isoforms. The elevated hCG can cause hyperthyroidism.

What are the thyroid function test changes during pregnancy?

Pregnancy brings many changes and the thyroid function tests are changed.

- During different trimesters, the thyroid function has a different normal value. However, we are not so sure about the exact value yet.
- During the first trimester, TSH is usually low due to elevated hCG.
- The total T3 and T4 are high due to the increased thyroid hormone-binding globulin (TBG). Usually we consider total T3 and T4 to be high if the number is greater than 1.5X the upper limit of nonpregnant women's normal value.

What are the symptoms of hyperthyroidism during pregnancy?

Many of the nonspecific symptoms associated with pregnancy are similar to those associated with hyperthyroidism, including but not limited to tachycardia, heat intolerance, increased perspiration, anxiety, hand tremor, and weight loss despite a normal or increased appetite. Specific findings such as goiter and ophthalmopathy suggest Graves' hyperthyroidism. The ophthalmopathy might be relieved during pregnancy.

Severe hyperthyroidism, if untreated can cause many complications:
- Spontaneous abortion
- Premature labor
- Low birth weight
- Stillbirth
- Preeclampsia
- Heart failure

How is the diagnosis of hyperthyroidism made during pregnancy?

If the patient has significant symptoms of hyperthyroidism (see above), although they are not specific, I would check the full panel of her

thyroid function. The medical society recommends doctors check TSH first and then if abnormal check FT4 and/or total T4, and if abnormal then check FT3 and/or total T3 in order to save money. However, this is another example of a recommendation from a "university professor" sitting in the office making recommendations. The sequential testing causes the patient to wait, delayed diagnosis, delayed treatment and more visits and results in increased cost.
I have many patients who are referred to me because they have low TSH.

When thyroid function tests indicate hyperthyroidism, I go ahead and order thyroid ultrasound and TSI testing. Thyroid ultrasound can show if the patient has nodules, possible Graves' disease or normal parenchyma. This information helps me to identify the cause of her hyperthyroidism.

I also have a non-pregnant patient who took a "thyroid supplement" which caused hyperthyroidism.

We do not do a radioactive iodine uptake and scan test although the dose is very low.

Why do some people feel the worsening of Graves' disease during the first trimester?

In my experience, the Graves' disease subsides during pregnancy. However, in the first trimester, the increasing of hCG cause the production of thyroid hormones. Therefore, in the first trimester, some patients might feel a worsening of their Graves' disease.

I have Graves' disease. Do I have to worry about my fetus having Graves' disease?

As we know the TSI passes the placenta and causes fetus to have hyperthyroidism although in my experience Graves' disease subsidizes. I still recommend having your TSI monitored. If your TSI is three times above normal, you need to be followed closely by your high-risk obstetrician,

How do you decide to treat or not to treat?

First, certainly, I would decide if the hyperthyroidism is severe enough to require treatment. Sometimes it is very hard to decide since the symptoms of hyperthyroidism are not specific.

Second, I try my best to identify the cause. Based on the cause, I make the decision jointly with the obstetrician and the patient.

How do you treat hyperthyroidism during pregnancy?

Again, I emphasize the cause of hyperthyroidism.
- Subclinical hyperthyroidism caused by elevated hCG: I usually just monitor and recommend no treatment.
- Overt hyperthyroidism caused by severely elevated hCG. I would not treat most cases, but I would treat if the patient has severe symptoms most likely caused by hyperthyroidism.
- My experience with Graves' patients is that the severity is lessened during pregnancy, Close monitoring is important, and I reduce medication if needed. I have quite a few Graves' disease patients who get into remission during pregnancy, therefore close monitoring is very important to reduce and even stop medication promptly.

- If the antithyroid medication was not high to start with, I just stop it as soon as the pregnancy is confirmed and check the thyroid function in 1-2 weeks.
- For hyperthyroidism caused by toxic nodules with severe hyperthyroidism, we recommend medication. Current recommendation is to use propylthiouracil in the first trimester and then switch to methimazole.
- Radioactive iodine is certainly not recommended at any stage of pregnancy.
- I have never referred a hyperthyroidism patient to have surgery during pregnancy.

If a patient cannot tolerate both anti-thyroid medications, what do you recommend?

The good news is that it is a very rare situation. As I discussed before, in many patients with Graves' disease, the severity subsides during pregnancy. So far, I do not have any pregnant women who cannot tolerate anti-thyroid medications. If I have, I would follow the American Thyroid Association recommendation to refer to have surgery. The surgery ideally will be in the second trimester. Certainly, you need to see a high-risk pregnancy team.

I have Graves' disease and was treated with RAI (or surgery) before pregnancy. Should I check my thyroid stimulating immunoglobulin (TSI)?

The RAI and thyroid surgery will not get your TSI to go away. I think you should check your TSI at the beginning of your pregnancy. If it is high, then you need to follow it in the middle of pregnancy. TSI can go through the placenta and cause the fetus to have Graves' disease. Again, it is not common partly due to the fact that pregnancy reduces the immunity and reduces the antibody production.

My hyperthyroidism was diagnosed during pregnancy. What should I do before my next pregnancy?

I would do my best to treat your hyperthyroidism. In other words, I would recommend surgery or RAI in between the pregnancies.

Chapter 9. Thyroid Hormone Replacement Therapy

What is the goal of treatment?

The treatment for hyperthyroidism (surgery or RAI) cause hypothyroidism. Surgery for Graves' disease cause 100% to have hypothyroidism. I only have one patient who did not have hypothyroidism after RAI. Simply to say, you are made to have hypothyroidism from hyperthyroidism. We want to eliminate your symptoms and signs of hypothyroidism; restore your sense of wellbeing; and we want to get your thyroid function test results to normal. As you know thyroid hormone is very important to your cells and you to function properly

What is the rate of hypothyroidism (low thyroid) in the course of hyperthyroidism?

Most hyperthyroidism patients become hypothyroidism due to treatment like surgery or RAI.

I have patients with hyperthyroidism that gradually burns out becoming hypothyroidism.

I also have patients who have had hypothyroidism for 40 years and suddenly converted to hyperthyroidism (overactive thyroid). For these patients, we usually recommend having surgery or radioactive iodine to burn the thyroid. It is never a good idea to leave it alone and wait for it to become hypothyroidism again by itself.

The thyroid hormone is very important for your body to function properly, therefore the thyroid hormone needs to be replaced.

My thyroid function is normal. Do I need any treatment?

If your thyroid function is normal, theoretically you do not need any thyroid hormone replacement therapy.

What medications for thyroid replacement are available on the market?

Currently we have the following medications from which you can choose to replace your thyroid hormone:

- Generic levothyroxine (T4)
- Levothroid (T4)
- Levoxyl (T4)
- Synthroid (T4)
- Unithyroid (T4)
- Tirosint (T4)
- Armour thyroid (T4+T3)
- Nature-throid(T4+T3)
- NP thyroid(T4+T3)
- WP-thyroid
- Cytomel (T3)

Which is best?

The most appropriate for you is the best.

What are the most commonly used medications in your clinic?

The most common one I use is generic levothyroxine. I also have a sizable number of patients on the brand names Synthroid and Levoxyl (which has been temporarily discontinued). Some patients are on Armour thyroid, Nature-throid, and NP thyroid. Only a few patients are on Tirosint and Cytomel.

While T4 formulation is generally recommended and most patients are doing very well in line with the major professional society's recommendations, I am not afraid to use other non-T4 formulations, like desiccated thyroid and combination of T4, or T3 alone or in combination with T4. I make decisions based on lab tests, but I do not disregard how patients feel. More importantly, I look into my patients' life and current medications because these two are the major factors in interpreting the thyroid function tests.

Is brand name Synthroid (other brand names in other areas) better than generic?

Theoretically, brand name Synthroid is better. It is more stable since it is manufactured by one manufacturer. Generic levothyroxine is manufactured by many different manufacturers. Even if you get it from the same pharmacy, it may be coming from different manufacturers.

However, for most people the variations introduced are not because of the different manufacturers. It is because they take their medication at different times and may even forget to take it. The most important thing is to take thyroid medication consistently.

If your insurance pays for it or other brand names, I do not have a problem starting patients on Synthroid.

Can I take other brand names instead of Synthroid?

I do not have any problems for my patients to start on any brand if their insurance pays for the other brand names. I have a few patients on Levoxyl but it has temporarily been discontinued. Synthroid is always present in my area of the country.

Can I be allergic to thyroid medication?

95

You should not be allergic to thyroid hormone itself but maybe to the "fillers" of the pill.

What "fillers" are present in Synthroid pill?

Acacia, confectioner's sugar (contains corn starch), lactose monohydrate, magnesium stearate, povidone, and talc. Different doses of medication also contain different coloring materials.

What is acacia? Could I be allergic to it?

Acacia is used to make the shape of the pill. It comes from shrubs and wood. Some people are allergic to it. If you have an allergy to tree pollens you might have an allergy to acacia, too.

I am lactose intolerant, and I saw Synthroid has lactose in it. Can I still take it?

The amount of lactose in the pill is very, very low. You should not have a problem taking it. However, there is a report that some patients might be allergic to it. Then you should not take it.

What is povidone? Is it toxic?

Povidone is a polymerized form of vinylpyrolidone, which is a white hygroscopic powder that is easily soluble in water and used as a dispersing and suspending agent in drugs like Synthroid.

It seems safe and I have not seen any research about allergies to povidone. People can have a mild or severe allergy to povidone-iodine which is used as skin disinfectant.

What is talc? Is it cancer causing?

Talc is a naturally occurring mineral mined from the earth that is composed of magnesium, silicon, oxygen, and hydrogen. Chemically, talc is a hydrous magnesium silicate with a chemical formula of Mg3Si4O10(OH)2.

Talc has many uses in cosmetics and other personal care products, in food such as rice and chewing gum, and in the manufacturing of tablets.

Asbestos, the cousin of talc, is a cancer-causing agent. There is no evidence to show that talc causes cancer or allergies. In recent Johnson Johnson lawsuit, the plaintiffs claimed that the baby powder was contaminated by asbestos.

Synthroid comes in different colors. What are the color agents in the pill?

Synthroid has 12 different strengths (mcg) with 12 different colors.

Table. Synthroid tablet color and additives.

Strength (mcg)	Color additive(s)
25	orange--FD&C Yellow No. 6 Aluminum Lake
50	white------None
75	violet----FD&C Red No. 40 Aluminum Lake, and FD&C Blue No. 2 Aluminum Lake
88	olive------FD&C Blue No. 1 Aluminum Lake, FD&C Yellow No. 6 Aluminum Lake, D&C Yellow No. 10 Aluminum Lake
100	yellow---D&C Yellow No. 10 Aluminum Lake, FD&C Yellow No. 6 Aluminum Lake

Strength (mcg)	Color additive(s)
112	rose--D&C Red No. 27 & 30 Aluminum Lake
125	brown-FD&C Yellow No. 6 Aluminum Lake, FD&C Red No. 40 Aluminum Lake, FD&C Blue No. 1 Aluminum Lake
137	Turquoise-FD&C Blue No. 1 Aluminum Lake
150	blue-FD&C Blue No. 2 Aluminum Lake
175	lilac-FD&C Blue No. 1 Aluminum Lake, D&C Red No. 27 & 30 Aluminum Lake
200	pink-FD&C Red No. 40 Aluminum Lake
300	green-D&C Yellow No. 10 Aluminum Lake, FD&C Yellow No. 6 Aluminum Lake, FD&C Blue No. 1 Aluminum Lake

Is aluminum lake toxic?

Aluminum lake is aluminum oxide. It is believed to be nontoxic.

Can I be allergic to dyes?

Yes, it is possible. If suspected, you can try the dosage of 50 ug which does not have coloring agents. I use this as a base to make different doses. The following is my scheme to make different doses;

- 25 ug: ½ tab daily
- 50 ug: 1 tab daily
- 75 ug: 1 and ½ tabs daily
- 88 ug: 5 days of 2 tabs daily, and 2 days of 1 tab daily
- 100 ug: 2 tabs daily
- 112 ug: 6 days of 2 tabs daily and one day of 3.5 tabs
- 125 ug: 2.5 tabs daily
- 137 ug:3 tabs daily for 6 daily and 1 tab for one day
- 150 ug: 3 tabs daily
- 175 ug:3.5 tabs daily
- 200 ug: 4 tabs daily
- 250 ug: 5 tabs daily
- 300 ug: 6 tabs daily

Why are colors added to the pills?

I have no ideal. I think the manufacturers might want to help patients to identify the pills because there are so many different doses.

What is the color scheme for other T4 brands?

Most of them use the same color scheme, but there are some differences.

Strength (ug)	Levothroid (Actavis)	Levoxyl (Pfizer)	Synthroid (Abbvie)	Unithroid (Watson)
25	orange	orange	orange	peach
50	white	white	white	white
75	violet	purple	violet	purple
88	mint green	olive	olive	olive
100	yellow	yellow	yellow	yellow
112	rose	rose	rose	rose
125	brown	brown	brown	tan
137	deep blue	dark blue	turquoise	Not available
150	blue	blue	blue	blue
175	lilac	turquoise	lilac	lilac
200	pink	pink	pink	pink
300	green	green	green	green

Is the gel form Tirosint better?

It is believed that the gel form Tirosint has better absorption. Patients with atrophic gastritis, patients taking anti-acid medications, or patients with a history of gastric bypass surgery could benefit from this due to absorption issues. I do not worry about this too much, I usually just increase the dose. The gel form is more expensive. If your insurance will pay for it and you believe it works better for you, I do not have a problem prescribing it.

I have patients who have malabsorption and I have prescribed 500-1000 ug of levothyroxine. I wanted to try Tirosint but was not able to get their insurance to pay for it.

What fillers does Tirosint have?

Inactive ingredients: gelatin, glycerin, and water.
People might have an allergic reaction to gelatin, but usually not to glycerin.

Does Tirosint have color coding?

No, Tirosint does not have color coding on the gel. If you are allergic to color agents, this version might be a good option for you. However, if your insurance doesn't pay for it or it is too expensive for you, you can use my scheme to form a different dose with colorless 50 ug pills.

On the boxes, the color coding is as follows.

Strength (ug)	Color on the box
13	green
25	peach
50	white
100	purple
112	yellow
125	brown
150	blue

Does Tirosint cause fewer allergic reactions?

Yes. Tirosint has fewer fillers and no coloring agents added. If you are looking for "pure" thyroid hormone replacement, this is the purest.

I have patients who also claimed to have an allergic reaction to it. Presumably they are allergic to gelatin. Many vaccines also have gelatin. If you are allergic to vaccines then you might be allergic to Tirosint, but vaccines have more allergens in them.

How are Tirosint capsules supplied?

They are supplied as follows: Boxes of 56 capsules, consisting of eight blisters with seven capsules each.

What is the best time to take T4 formulations like generic levothyroxine, Synthroid, Levoxyl, Levothroid, Unithroid, or Tirosint?

It is recommended to take them early in the morning on an empty stomach. Ideally, take it 60 minutes before you drink anything except water, eat, or take any other medications.

However, most of my patients are not able to do that. I usually ask my patients to put the medication and a cup of water on their nightstand the night before and, as soon as they open their eyes, pop in the medication with a cup of water. During the night, you lose a lot of water, so it is good for you to drink a cup of water when you wake up.

Can I take T4 formulations like generic levothyroxine, Synthroid, Levoxyl, Levothroid, Unithroid, or Tirosint at night?

I have patients who cannot take it early in the morning, so I ask them to take it before going to bed. I urge them to not eat any snacks after dinner. Bedtime and dinner should be at least four hours apart.

What should I do if I forget a day?

It is best not to forget, but life happens, so if you forget, I recommend you double it the next day.

Do you have any options for my son who is 16 years old? He never remembers to take his meds and I cannot be after him every day to take them.

Your son is not alone. Lots of teens are not good at taking medications. They either forget, do not want to take it, or wake up too late and rush. It is very challenging for teens to take thyroid medication.

I recommend my patients choose one day each week and take seven pills all at once. It is not ideal but at least you know they consistently get taken.

I have malabsorption. What options do I have?

Tirosint may be better for you if your insurance will pay for it. Otherwise, I would just increase your dose.

However, I have patients who have such severe malabsorption that we must give intravenous levothyroxine periodically and their insurance usually balks at paying for it.

I have Crohn's disease. Do you have any recommendations for me?

Crohn's disease is an inflammatory bowel disease. It can be very challenging with flare ups and changes in absorption rates in the body. You can try Tirosint which has a better absorption rate. The key issue is to check your thyroid function more often.

I am also taking iron and calcium supplements. Any extra precautions?

Iron and calcium affect thyroid medication absorption significantly. I recommend taking your calcium or iron pills at least four hours after taking your thyroid medication. If you take your thyroid medication in the morning, then I recommend you take iron or calcium at supper or at night.

I am also taking osteoporosis medication called bisphosphonates-like Actonel (risedronate), Fosamax (alendronate), Boniva (ibandronate), Pamidronate. Can I take my thyroid hormone with these medications?

These medications also require you to take them early in the morning on an empty stomach and then wait 60 minutes before you eat or drink anything else except water.

Since these medications are usually taken once a week or once a month, I am not particularly worried about these.

If you take your thyroid medication and osteoporosis medication together, it might affect the thyroid medication absorption. Since T4 formulations (generic levothyroxine, Synthroid, Levoxyl, Levothroid, Unithroid, or Tirosint) come with half-life of seven days, one day of lower absorption will not affect your blood thyroid level too much. Your thyroid hormone level will be stable.

If you do not want to take them together, you can also omit your thyroid hormone on the day you are taking the bisphosphonate and then double your thyroid medication the next day.

However, if you are newly starting your bisphosphonate, I recommend having your thyroid function checked in six weeks and adjusting your dose as needed.

I am also taking acid reflux / stomach medications - H pump inhibitors, like Nexium (esoprazole), Omeprazole, Pantoprazole, Lansoprazole, Dexilant (dexlansoprazole), or Aciphex (rabeprazole) medications. My doctors tell me to take them on an empty stomach. What should I do?

These medications might reduce thyroid medication absorption, but most studies say NO. The good news is that your doctor can always increase the thyroid medication dose as needed. I first let my patients take their thyroid medication with these medications together on an empty stomach to see if we can get their thyroid level stable.

Another option is to take the thyroid medication at night. However, these patients are also taking other medications at night which might affect their thyroid medication absorption. It is better to take them together in the morning.

I have patients who like to take thyroid medication 30 minutes before taking these mentioned medications. This option is also acceptable. The key issue is consistency.

Certainly, if you start later you will need to check your thyroid function in four to six weeks after you have started on H pump inhibitors to make sure you are taking sufficient thyroid medication.

I am taking antacids, what should I pay attention to?

If you are taking antacids like aluminum hydroxide, magnesium hydroxide, Alka-seltzer, Pepto-Bismol, Maalox, Mylanta (aluminum hydroxide/magnesium hydroxide), Rolaids, or Tums, these medications should be taken at least four hours after thyroid medication. I strongly recommend taking your thyroid medication early in the morning on an empty stomach with a cup of room temperature or warm water.

If you are taking your antacids periodically, you really need to take your thyroid medication first, take it consistently early in the morning on an empty stomach, and wait 45-60 minutes before you eat, drink, or take anything else. These antacids should not be taken within four hours of thyroid medications.

I am taking Carafate for my stomach ulcer. I heard this medication can affect thyroid medication absorption. What should I do?

It is true that Carafate reduces thyroid medication absorption. This medication might be taken four times a day and needs to be taken one hour before a meal. In this situation, I recommend taking your thyroid medication 30 minutes before taking Carafate with a cup of warm water. Close monitoring and adjusting thyroid medication is strongly recommended.

What other medications should I pay attention to while taking thyroid medication?

If you are taking any of the following medications, you should take them at least four hours apart from thyroid medication. Consistency is the key. Let your thyroid doctor know so the dose can be adjusted.

- Cholestyramine - cholesterol medication.
- Colesevelam - cholesterol medication.
- Selevemer - lower phosphorus in renal failure patients.
- Raloxifene (Evista) - breast cancer prevention and treating osteoporosis.

There are certainly many other medications which might affect thyroid medication absorption. Keep taking the medications four hours apart if you can.

I was told that I cannot take my thyroid medication with coffee. However, I always rush in the morning. There is no way that I can wait 60 minutes before I drink my coffee. Are you sure I absolutely cannot drink coffee?

Life is complicated as you described and taking thyroid medication certainly makes it more complicated. I am very liberal: If you are willing to promise that you drink the same coffee at the same time every day, I will let you try. We can always adjust your thyroid medication dose.

Another option is to take your thyroid medication at night. After dinner you are not supposed to eat snacks for at least four hours.

I cannot wait 60 minutes before I eat my breakfast. What should I do?

Milk and soy products, coffee and other fibers all affect thyroid medication absorption. As I recommended before, prepare a cup of water on your nightstand the night before. As soon as you open your eyes, you can pop in your thyroid medication. After you get washed and dressed, 30 minutes might have passed. This is not 60 minutes as recommended, but it will be acceptable.

I also have patients taking their thyroid medication when they wake up in the middle of night or early morning. You are allowed to take it at that time.

Whatever you do, if you can do it consistently it is not a big deal. We can always adjust your dose.

How do you decide which dose to start?

I use the information of the patient's weight, lean body mass, pregnancy status, cause of hypothyroidism (RAI or surgery), degree of TSH elevation, age, history of cardiovascular disease, and other conditions including the presence of cardiac disease. The most important thing is to follow up and adjust your medication. It is very important to start right, but more importantly to adjust and take your medication correctly and consistently.

I swear that I feel better when I am on Armour thyroid. My former endocrinologist did not believe me. Do you believe me?

I believe you, and I have 20% of my patients who like to take a desiccated thyroid product like Armour thyroid.

The thyroid gland is complicated. The thyroid gland secretes a variety of iodinated and non-iodinated molecules that collectively play important roles during our prenatal and adult lives. We do not understand them yet. When I was an Endocrine Fellow at Washington University, School of Medicine, I had a fellow classmate who did research on calcitonin. He claimed that replacement of calcitonin affects feelings of well-being.

My approach to this request is to keep an open mind. I acknowledge that a T4 formulation like levothyroxine is the mainstream supplement and it is very easy to take. Most patients are doing very well on this. I let patients try other formulations if they are not happy about their current medication. I do let patients know that there are many reasons which might cause them to not feel well that we cannot fix with thyroid medications. I also let my patients know that sometimes we will have to use desiccated thyroid two times a day due to high levels of T3 in it. The dose difference between each batch may be larger even from the same manufacturer, and sometimes it is very difficult to have a right dose. Also, the T4, T3 and other molecules might also vary from batch to batch. Desiccated thyroid also requires a lab test that is sometimes difficult for a non-specialist to interpret.

The manufacturer also advises that a potential risk of product contamination with porcine and bovine viral or other adventitious agents cannot be ruled out.

What is Armour thyroid anyway?

Armour Thyroid for oral use is a natural preparation derived from porcine thyroid glands. They provide 38 mcg levothyroxine (T4) and 9 mcg liothyronine (T3) per grain of thyroid (equivalent of 60 mg).

What is WP thyroid or Nature-throid?

They are two other products from desiccated pig thyroid. I treat them the same as Armour thyroid, however the dose forms are slightly different.

What is the dose equivalent between desiccated thyroid and T4 preparations like levothyroxine?

Usually, I start 100 ug of levothyroxine converted to 60 mg (one grain) of Armour thyroid or 65 mg (one grain) of WP thyroid or Nature-throid.

The Armour thyroid and NP thyroid have a dose increment of 15 mg (equivalent to levothyroxine 25 ug).

The WP thyroid and Nature-throid have dose increments of 16.25 mg equivalent to levothyroxine 25 ug..

Table of the dose conversions between commonly used thyroid replacement preparations.

Levothyroxine Mcg	Armour grain(mg)	WP thyroid grain(mg)	Nature-throid grain(mg)
25	¼(15)	¼(16.25)	¼(16.25)
50	½(30)	½(32.5)	½(32.5)
75		¾(48.75)	¾(48.75)
88			
100	1(60)	1(65)	1(65)
112			
125		1.25(81.25)	1/25(81.25)
137			
150	1.5(90)	1.5(97.5)	1.5(97.5)
175		1.75(113.75)	1.75(113.75)
200	2(120)	2(130)	2(130)
			2.25(146.25)
			2.5(162.5)
300	3(180)		3(195)
	4(240)		4(260)
	5(300)		5(325)

Please note this is just a starting point. Everyone is different. You need to closely monitor your thyroid function and get your dose adjusted accordingly.

What are the inactive ingredients in the pill?

The inactive ingredients are calcium stearate, dextrose, microcrystalline cellulose, sodium starch glycolate, and opadry white.

Can I have an allergy to natural desiccated thyroid?

Yes, you can.

Can I take my Armour thyroid or other desiccated thyroid at night?

Theoretically it is okay to take it at night. The thyroid effect in cells needs a few hours to work. However, I still have patients complaining about it affecting their sleep. My point is that you can try it and if it does not affect your sleep, you can take it at bedtime.

I am on a thyroid supplement. Do I need to take extra iodine?

No, you do not. You already are being supplemented with iodine, a product of the thyroid hormone.

I am on a thyroid supplement. Do I need to take a selenium supplement?

Selenium helps you to convert T4 to the active hormone T3. However, most people do not have a selenium deficiency and you do not need to take it. If you want to take it, it is acceptable, and it might help you. However, if you take too much, it can cause toxicity.

My TSH is low. Why did my doctor reduce my thyroid medication?

TSH is like a thermostat. It works like an internal monitor of your thyroid hormone. If your thyroid hormone level is too high, then TSH is going to be reduced. The opposite is true also. If your thermostat ramps up it means the temperature at your house is too low. If the TSH is too high, it means your thyroid hormone level is too low. That is why when your TSH is low your doctor will lower your thyroid medication; if your TSH is too high, your doctor will increase your medication.

Just remember, the TSH level is always opposite to your thyroid hormone level. The premise is that you have a normal pituitary gland.

I heard that taking thyroid medication can help me lose weight. Can I take more?

It is really a bad idea to take more thyroid medication to lose weight. Too much thyroid medication may cause atrial fibrillation which will increase your risk for a stroke. Too much thyroid medication can also cause osteoporosis. These are the two most serious long term side effects. Other side effects are anxiety, sweaty, insomnia, diarrhea, and "irritable bowel syndrome".

Why is my FT4 always elevated and TSH is normal?

This usually occurs with the following situation:
Most patients are being treated with T4 (levothyroxine, Synthroid, Levoxyl, etc). The medication usually is being absorbed within four hours and can have a peak at blood. If you check your blood two to four hours after you take your medication, your blood value of T4 might be higher than normal.

Do I need to reduce my dose if FT4 is high?

No, I adjust your medication based on many factors.

As we can see from the previous question, T4 will peak in two to four hours after taking the medication. You certainly do not need to reduce your medication if this is the case. I usually look at the full panel of thyroid function and your symptoms and signs. If your TSH is suppressed and you have some signs of overactive thyroid, certainly we need to reduce your dose.

My FT3 is always low. What are the reasons?

I assume your TSH and FT4 are normal. Here are some of the reasons:

- You had a total thyroidectomy or RAI, which means your thyroid doesn't work at all. Since thyroid is responsible to produce 20% of T3, now you do not have it.
- You might be taking some medications which can suppress deiodinase which are the enzymes responsible to convert T4 to T3.
- You might have low activity of deiodinase gene function.

What are the medications that might inhibit the function of deiodinase?

There is a long list of medications which might inhibit the conversion of T4 to T3. Here are a few common ones:

- Steroids
- Beta blockers, especially propranolol. Other commonly used beta blockers are atenolol, metoprolol, labetalol, Coreg.
- Amiodarone (medication for irregular heart beat). Amiodarone can cause a range of thyroid problems.
- Lithium (mood stabilizer). Lithium can cause a spectrum of thyroid issues.

What are the common conditions which might inhibit the function of deiodinase?

Some conditions and disease status can also inhibit deiodinase, reducing T4 to T3 conversion:
- Very sick
- Lots of stress
- Lots of inflammation
- Starvation/deprivation
- Selenium deficiency

What can I do if my T3 is low?

There are many options. I make the decision depending on the patient's clinical comorbidities and symptoms. If you are relatively healthy, TSH is still normal, but you still have lots of hypothyroidism symptoms, I might increase your thyroid medication dose or add a low dose T3 into the regimen. If you are not on desiccated thyroid. I might let you try.

My doctor changes my dose every time I have my lab test. What should I do?

You are not alone. I have quite a few patients who are referred to me for unstable thyroid. They have tried every dose of thyroid medication. I recommend you see an Endocrinologist if this describes your situation.

I take my medication everyday consistently. Why does my thyroid level still change with every lab test?

Both you and your doctor should realize that thyroid hormone absorption can be affected by many foods you are eating and many medications especially calcium and iron you are taking. You might also want to make sure you do not have absorption problems like celiac disease or Crohn's disease.

Some patients are very sensitive to thyroid hormones. I recommend my patients to strictly take their medication consistently and to try a brand-name preparation like Synthroid. If they are taking a calcium or iron supplement (many multiple vitamins have both), I ask them to take such supplements at least four hours after. Taking other supplement consistently is also very important, since these supplements can affect thyroid hormone absorption even four hours after.

I take my medication everyday consistently and correctly. Why is my thyroid function still low?

Occasionally, I have patients who needs a high dose of thyroid medication. The most common reason is that patient is not taking the medication correctly or often misses the medication. However, I trust my patients if they tell me that they are taking the medication correctly and consistently. These are the situations I have encountered:

- Patients have celiac disease. As we know, the risk for celiac disease is increased in patients with Graves' disease / Hashimoto's thyroiditis.
- Patients have short gut syndrome.
- Patients have history of gastric by-pass surgery.
- Patients have severe inflammatory bowel disease, like Crohn's disease.
- Patients have high level of proteinuria.
- Patients are taking some medications like efavirenz, cimetidine, sodium valproate, etc.
- Patients have liver hemangioendothelioma (not everyone). Some tumors were found to have over express type 3 iodothyronine deiodinase activity and increased catalysis of

the conversion of thyroxine (T4) to reverse triiodothyronine (T3), and of T3 to diidothyronine (T2) by this enzyme.

What is pseudomalabsorption of levothyroxine?

I have a patient who came to me for uncontrolled thyroid. She had Graves' disease and was treated with RAI many years ago. When she came to see me, she was taking 500 ug daily but her TSH was still over 50-100. Initially she said she took her medications consistently. Later she admitted that she had to stop periodically because she did not feel well with anxiety, diarrhea, poor sleep, etc., with the symptoms of hyperthyroidism.

So, what happened was that initially she was not taking her medication consistently, then her doctor increased her medication every time to the level which caused her to have an overactive level of thyroid hormone. She took it a few days and then stopped or did not take it at all for very long periods of time.

The patient did not have an absorption problem but presented as a malabsorption problem. We call this kind of situation a pseudomalabsoption of levothyroxine. In my experience, this happens often to young moms. They are so busy taking care of the baby and other needs in their lives and forget their medication. Therefore, I always try my best to make sure that the patient is taking the medication consistently and correctly before I raise the dose.

I have hypothyroidism (underactive thyroid) treated with thyroid medication for 40 years, and now my doctor said that I have hyperthyroidism (overactive thyroid). Is this possible?

The exact cause and disease process are not yet very clear. Some patients have two kinds of antibody. One antibody can block the thyrotropin receptor and then cause hypothyroidism (Hashimoto's

116

thyroiditis), and one antibody can stimulate the thyrotropin receptor and then cause hyperthyroidism (overactive thyroid, Hashimoto's thyrotoxicosis). I have had quite a few patients like you who have had long standing hypothyroidism and then converted to hyperthyroidism. In such cases, I just treat as hyperthyroidism. Eventually I treated them with surgery or radioactive iodine.

Chapter 10. Hyperthyroidism and Diet

Can diet therapy cure my hyperthyroidism?

As we can see from Chapter 1, there are many reasons that might lead to hyperthyroidism. Diet can have significant effect on thyroid function, but if you have moderate to severe hyperthyroidism, please do not rely on diet only to cure your hyperthyroidism.

Hyperthyroidism is a serious condition and you need to see your doctor and follow your doctor's recommendations.

Should I eat more food rich in iodine?

No, you should not. Iodine is crucial to make thyroid hormone. If you eat more iodine, like when you put more gas on a fire, your hyperthyroidism might get worse.

Should I stay away from iodine rich food?

Before your hyperthyroidism is controlled, you should stay away from iodine rich food. For iodine rich food, please read Chapter 4 of this book, or my other books *Thyroid Nodule, Hashimoto's thyroiditis Hypothyroidism Fatigue*. Please also review the low panel of the front cover.

Do I have to stay away from iodine rich food for the rest of my life?

NO, as soon as your hyperthyroidism is under control, you can eat whatever you want. Hyperthyroidism can be controlled by medication, radioactive iodine or surgery.

What kind of diet should I follow?

No diet can cure your hyperthyroidism. However, there are a few things you can consider:

- Numerous patients have significant weight loss. If you do not like the weight loss, you are okay to eat a high protein and high carb diet.
- 10% of hyperthyroidism patients have weight gain. If this is the case for you, you certainly need to practice caution about your portion size and meal frequency. You are recommended to reduce your carbs and fat intake. You should eat more vegetables. However, this is easy to say but hard to do. The increased appetite is hard to deal with at this condition.
- You are recommended to eat a high fiber diet. Thyroid hormones are recycled, in other words, thyroid hormones are secreted into the intestine and then reabsorbed. If you are eating a high fiber diet, then less thyroid hormone will be reabsorbed.
- You are recommended to eat more cruciferous vegetables for two reasons: 1) vegetables have more fibers which reduce your intestinal thyroid hormone recycles; 2) cruciferous vegetables have compounds to reduce the iodine getting into the thyroid cells to make thyroid hormone.
- Some examples of cruciferous vegetables are: broccoli, cauliflower, cassava, bok choy, bamboo shoots, collard greens, kale, and mustard.

I have Graves' disease. What else should I pay more attention to in my diet?

Graves' disease is an autoimmune disease which can travel with other autoimmune diseases. It is reported that the celiac disease rate is increased in patients with Graves' disease. If you are suspected to have celiac disease you need to be on a gluten free diet.

Diet has been suggested to be associated with autoimmune disease, but there is no concrete association yet. Generally, I recommend not drinking milk or eating dairy before your hyperthyroidism is controlled. Milk and dairy products also have too much iodine.

Should I eat more soy and soy products?

It is not a bad idea to eat more soy and soy products for the following reasons: 1) soy has chemicals which can reduce the iodine getting into the thyroid cells to make more thyroid hormones, 2) soy has good plant proteins which help supplement healthy protein for your body to prevent too much weight loss. Some people believe it is not a good idea to eat soy due to its possible effect on the thyroid. There is yet no clinical trial to settle this controversy.

Should I take an iron supplement?

Hyperthyroidism increases metabolism. Everything in your body is being consumed faster. It is not a bad idea to take some iron supplements for the following reasons: 1) the iron deficiency anemia rate is increased in patients with hyperthyroidism; 2) iron actually reduces the thyroid hormone recycle, as we stated above. Thyroid hormone is being secreted into the intestine and being reabsorbed. Iron actually can reduce the thyroid hormone recycles and iodine reabsorption; 3) hyperthyroidism can cause loose stool or diarrhea, while iron supplements cause the opposite.

121

Should I take calcium and vitamin D supplements?

It is a little more complicated than an iron supplement.
Hyperthyroidism also increases bone metabolism in a small group of patients who have hypercalcemia. If this is the case, you might not need to have a calcium supplement. However, if your calcium is normalized, then you should take some calcium and vitamin D to rebuild your bones.

Calcium also reduces your thyroid hormone recycles which can help relieve your hyperthyroidism.

Should I take other vitamins?

Since hyperthyroidism increases metabolism which might cause other vitamin deficiencies, it is not a bad idea to take some vitamin supplement. Just make sure not to take multiple vitamins with iodine before you have controlled your hyperthyroidism.

It is really a good idea to take more vitamin B which is very important for metabolism. Folic acid is also very important in making blood.

Should I take some selenium supplement?

Selenium is believed to have a function in immune regulation. Hyperthyroidism increases the consumption anyway. It is okay to take some supplement. As I stated elsewhere, do not take too much. It might have some toxicity.

Should I use more spices?

Spices like hot pepper you might need to void before your hyperthyroidism is being controlled. They have many good nutrients, but they make you feel hot and might increase your metabolism and your hyperthyroidism already has increased your metabolism.

Should I take some herbs for my hyperthyroidism?

It is not a good idea. In Ancient China, it was remarkable for ancient Chinese to figure out how to treat goiter with some Chinese herbs / seaweed, but goiter with hyperthyroidism is not a condition which can be treated with Chinese herbs.

I am always tired. Can I take more turmeric?

Turmeric is believed to have anti-inflammatory effects which might be helpful for your hyperthyroidism. The real effect is not known.

.

www.ingramcontent.com/pod-product-compliance
Lightning Source LLC
Chambersburg PA
CBHW060610200326
41521CB00007B/723